Basics of

Kidney, Renal Disease, Fluid, Electrolyte and Acid–Base Balance

for Students of

- Nursing • Paramedical Courses and
- Allied Health Sciences

Basics of

Kidney, Renal Disease, Fluid, Electrolyte and Acid–Base Balance

for Students of

- **Nursing** • **Paramedical Courses and**
- **Allied Health Sciences**

Editor

R Kasi Visweswaran
MD, DM (Nephrology), FRCP (Edin)

Consultant in Nephrology
Ananthapuri Hospitals and Research Institute
Thiruvananthapuram, Kerala

Ex-Professor of Nephrology
Medical College
Thiruvananthapuram, Kerala

Visiting Professor
Pushpagiri Medical College
Thiruvalla, Kerala

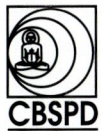

CBSPD

CBS Publishers & Distributors Pvt Ltd

New Delhi • Bengaluru • Chennai • Kochi • Kolkata • Lucknow • Mumbai
Hyderabad • Jharkhand • Nagpur • Patna • Pune • Uttarakhand

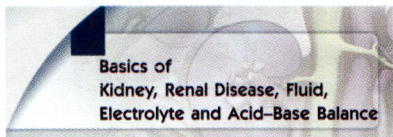

**Basics of
Kidney, Renal Disease, Fluid,
Electrolyte and Acid–Base Balance**

ISBN: 978-93-86217-58-5

Copyright © Author and Publisher

First Edition: 2017

Reprint: 2024

Published by Satish Kumar Jain and produced by Varun Jain for

CBS Publishers & Distributors Pvt Ltd

4819/XI Prahlad Street, 24 Ansari Road, Daryaganj, New Delhi 110 002, India.
Ph: 23289259, 23266861   Website: www.cbspd.com

e-mail: delhi@cbspd.com; cbspubs@airtelmail.in.

Corporate Office: 204 FIE, Industrial Area, Patparganj, Delhi 110 092
Ph: 4934 4934   Fax: 4934 4935   e-mail: publishing@cbspd.com; publicity@cbspd.com

Branches

• **Bengaluru:** Seema House 2975, 17th Cross, K.R. Road, Banasankari 2nd Stage,
  Bengaluru 560 070, Karnataka
  Ph: +91-80-26771678/79   Fax: +91-80-26771680   e-mail: bangalore@cbspd.com
• **Chennai:** 7, Subbaraya Street, Shenoy Nagar, Chennai 600 030, Tamil Nadu, India
  Ph: +91-44-26680620/26681266   Fax: +91-44-42032115   e-mail: chennai@cbspd.com
• **Kochi:** 42/1325, 1326, Power House Road, Opp KSEB, Power House, Ernakulam 682 018,
  Kochi, Kerala, India
  Ph: +91-484-4059061-65, 67   Fax: +91-484-4059065   e-mail: kochi@cbspd.com
• **Kolkata:** 147, Hind Ceramics Compound, 1st Floor, Nilgunj Road, Belghoria, Kolkata-700056,
  West Bengal, India
  Ph: +033-25633055, 033-25633056   e-mail: kolkata@cbspd.com
• **Lucknow:** Basement, Khushnuma Complex, 7 Meerabai Marg (Behind Jawahar Bhawan),
  Lucknow-226001, UP, India

  Ph: +91-522-4000032   e-mail: tiwari.lucknow@cbspd.com
• **Mumbai:** PWD Shed, Gala no 25/26, Ramchandra Bhatt Marg, Next to JJ Hospital
  Gate no. 2, Opp. Union Bank of India Noorbaug, Mumbai-400009, Maharashtra, India
  Ph: 022-66661880/89   e-mail: mumbai@cbspd.com

Representatives

| • **Hyderabad** | 0-9885175004 | • **Jharkhand** | 0-9811541605 | • **Nagpur** | 0-8692091830 |
| • **Patna** | 0-9334159340 | • **Pune** | 0-9664372571 | • **Uttarakhand** | 0-9716462459 |

Printed at: Sri Prints and Sales, Delhi, India

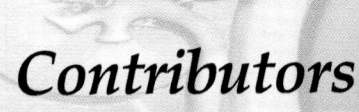

Contributors

Dhanya Binu MD
Assistant Professor, Department of Pathology

G Vijayalakshmi MD
Professor, Department of Anatomy

John Joseph MS, MCh (Pediatric surgery)
Associate Professor, Department of Pediatric Surgery

Jose Paul MD, DM (Nephrology)
Associate Professor, Department of Nephrology

Leni Kumar Joseph MD
Assistant Professor, Department of Pediatrics

Manu G Krishnan MD, DM (Nephrology)
Assistant Professor, Department of Nephrology

R. Hema MS, MCh (Pediatric Surgery)
Professor, Department of Pediatric Surgery

R Kasi Visweswaran MD, DM (Nephrology) FRCP (Edin)
Visiting Professor, Department of Nephrology

Reena Thomas MD, DM (Nephrology)
Professor and Head, Department of Nephrology

Satheesh Balakrishnan MD, DM (Nephrology)
Assistant Professor, Department of Nephrology

Sushama Bai MD, DCH
Professor and Head, Department of Pediatrics

Terese Kochuvilayil SIC, MSc (Nursing)
Associate Professor-Cum-Head, Department of Medical Surgical Nursing

Vikram Gowda MD
Associate Professor, Department of Physiology

All contributors are current or former faculty members of Pushpagiri Institute of Medical Sciences, Thiruvalla, Kerala.

Foreword

I am happy to write the Foreword to the book entitled *Basics of Kidney, Renal Disease, Fluid, Eectrolyte and Acid–Base Balance* edited by Prof R Kasi Visweswaran with contributions from the teaching faculty of Pushpagiri Group of Institutions, Tiruvalla, Kerala.

It was a pleasure going through the book intended for nursing and technical staff of departments of nephrology and the various technology-oriented branches of a fully-fledged nephrology unit. Nephrology practice leans to a great extent on sophisticated technical support and accurate laboratory monitoring at all stages—starting from diagnosis and medical management through dialysis and renal transplantation. Post-transplant period also demands periodic examination and close monitoring to achieve good results. The need for a book which will give the theoretical basis of the various aspects met with in this specialty and instructions in a practical way will go a long way in improving the nephrology services in all secondary and tertiary care hospitals.

Even though renal diseases affect 20% of the population in some way or the other, compared to other specialities like cardiology and neurology, the number of nephrologists and nephrology centers is less. Prof Kasi Visweswaran belongs to the early group of nephrologists in the country, trained and encouraged by the doyens in Indian nephrology scene, Prof KS Chugh of PGI, Chandigarh.

Prof Kasi Visweswaran has held top posts in nephrology for over three decades in the government medical colleges at Kottayam and Trivandrum. He has vast experience in starting and nurturing full-fledged departments of nephrology. He has been a postgraduate teacher for DM nephrology, DNB nephrology and has visited many institutions inside and outside the country.

His contributions to medical books are wide, ranging from chapters on nephrology in textbooks of internal medicine, clinical medicine, nephrology and monographs in nephrology. He has contributed important chapters in popular international textbook *Comprehensive Clinical Nephrology*. He has been the editor of monographs in nephrology such as *Essentials of Nephrology and Urology, Essentials of Nephrology and Prescribing Drugs in Renal Diseases*. He is also a coeditor with Prof Claudio Ponticelli (Italy) of the book *Current Progress in Nephrology* to be published shortly. He has authored the book *Handbook of Fluid, Eectrolyte and Acid–Base Balance* being published by CBS Publishers & Distributors

A practical guide, including the necessary level of theoretical information and practical hands on details on several aspects of nursing, diet, dialysis, renal transplantation and follow-up, is required for all nurses, technicians, and other auxiliary staff of departments of nephrology. This necessity is greater at present when several medium and large institutions are coming up in India—in public, corporate and private sectors. The number of books catering to this section of health care workers, presented in a simple language and suitable for the conditions prevailing in the country is limited.

The practical details needed for the nursing, technical, paramedical and laboratory staff are given in a lucid language. In the initial chapters, the editor and his team of authors have considered the theoretical aspects in a clear and understandable format particularly for the students who have undergone only a short exposure to these topics before their clinical posting. Since the nurse is the person who actually administers the intravenous fluids, three important chapters which explain the practical aspects and principles of fluid administration are also included.

I recommend this book to be kept as a practical guide for all departments of nephrology where basic and advanced work is undertaken.

Prof KV Krishna Das

BSc, FRCP (Edin), FAMS, DTM&H (Edin)

Ex-Director and Professor of Medicine
Medical College, Thiruvananthapuram

Foreword

I am delighted to pen the Foreword to *Basics of Kidney, Renal Disease, Fluid, Electrolyte and Acid–Base Balance* edited by Prof R Kasi Visweswaran, esteemed and eminent nephrologist. The chapters in this book are scripted by faculty from Pushpagiri Institute of Medical Sciences and Research Centre. As patron of this renowned institute, I sincerely congratulate Prof Kasi Visweswaran and the entire team for this precious endeavour.

Kidney diseases form a major cause of morbidity, especially with chronic conditions like diabetes. Due to increased awareness, earlier diagnosis and improved treatment facilities, the number of patients with renal problems is zooming up. Like born teachers, Prof Kasi and his team members have shown their talent and maturity of thinking, stressing on the base level knowledge, which may not be that evident in many similar works.

Nurses working in dialysis units, intensive care rooms, and even general medical and surgical wards should be adept in principles of fluid and acid–base disorders. Expertise in this area, quintessential while dealing with both acute and chronic kidney diseases, have been stressed sufficiently. Nursing staff should be able to interpret investigatory reports and understand the principles of management. Observations made by them are, many a time, permit me to qualify, *superior* to those by duty doctors. Thus, this book would certainly enhance their capacity and empower them by honing the skills of nurses towards providing adequate and better patient care. The importance of proper diet has also been dealt with.

Nurses from India, particularly from Kerala, are valued in other countries for their dedication and commitment. Guidance provided by this book would certainly aid them in securing skilled employment. It is surely a keepsake for nursing professionals, both as reference manual and as a ready-reckoner while on duty.

The authors have used their knowledge and wisdom from long years of experience to innovate the presentation of the subject according to the need of the times. This book would bridge any gap existing in the training of nursing staff and students, in the day-to-day nursing care of kidney disease patients.

Let me wish and hope that this book will be of tremendous assistance for all those who seek to read it! After all "the eye does not see what the mind does not know".

Dr Thomas Mar Koorilos
Metropolitan Archbishop of Tiruvalla

Preface

Nephrology is a rapidly developing field. Treatment of diseases of the kidney involves the nurses, dialysis/transplant technicians and paramedical staff. Ancillary departments like dietetics, bioengineering, biochemistry, pathology, microbiology, immunology, medical sociology, medical records and engineering workshop have a great role to play in the smooth functioning of the department. Fundamental knowledge of the subject is necessary to deliver their individual skills in their chosen field effectively. A nurse administering a drug should be aware of the basic principles—how it acts, what the side effects are, and how they can be prevented. They should be aware of simple calculations for determining the rate of intravenous fluid administration, which type of IV fluid should be given for which condition and be aware of the complications during therapy. Since the nurse is available round the clock, she is the first point of contact for the patient when any event develops. Basic knowledge of the subject will help to grasp and assess the situation quickly before reporting to a doctor. The teaching is that "If you are aware of what you are doing, you can seldom go wrong". This is very true in medicine and treatment. The biomedical engineer or the technicians in the engineering workshop should be aware of the special needs in relation to water supply and power. The dialysis technicians and the nurses are the ones actually performing the dialysis based on instructions from the doctors. The transplant technicians, operation theater assistants and post-transplant ICU nurses also must have a basic idea about the principles and procedures undertaken. The fluid balance charting is a very important part of nephrology nursing more so in the post-transplant ICU.

This book has been prepared with this theme in mind. In order to know why a particular treatment is given for a particular disease, a basic knowledge of the disease and the treatment options should be known—not only to the person who prescribes but also the person who implements the same. All the chapters are contributed by senior and experienced faculty from the Pushpagiri group of Institutions, Tiruvalla, Kerala. An efficient, knowledgeable and dedicated nurse is always a great asset to the institution. The nurses from Kerala, have earned a name for themselves throughout the world. Many students studying for a nursing degree or diploma have an eye on overseas career, although a good number of them also opt to remain in the country to treat their own countrymen. Wherever, they are working, knowledge of fundamentals is necessary to remain head and shoulders above the others in terms of knowledge and skill.

I, on behalf of my coauthors and myself, wish that the book will fulfill this aim and dream.

R Kasi Visweswaran

Contents

1 *Section*

Kidneys and Common Kidney Diseases

Anatomy of Urinary Tract

G Vijayalakshmi

The urinary tract comprises the organs and structures that are concerned with the formation and elimination of urine from the body. It belongs to the excretory system. The waste products of metabolism, mainly the urea and the creatinine, are excreted from the body through urine.

The urinary tract consists of the following parts (Fig. 1.1a):

1. A pair of kidneys
2. A pair of ureters
3. Urinary bladder
4. Urethra

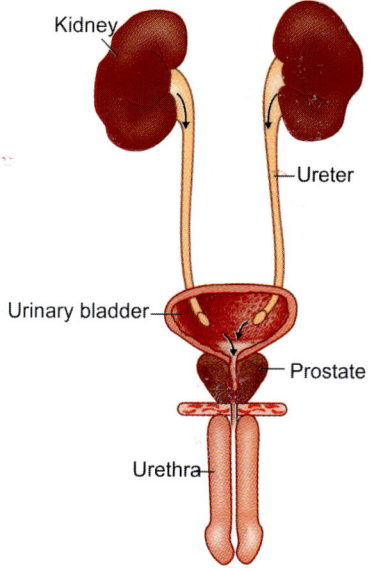

Fig. 1.1a: Urinary tract—male

Urine is formed in the kidneys through filtration of blood. It is conveyed through the ureters to the urinary bladder, which acts as a temporary storehouse. The bladder is emptied periodically. During micturition, the urine passes through the urethra and is discharged to the external environment. The urinary tract in the males and the females are the same except in the length and course of the urethra (Fig. 1.1b).

KIDNEYS

The kidneys are excretory organs that remove waste products of metabolism like urea, creatinine and uric acid from the body, and excrete them through urine. They also reabsorb the substances useful for the body from the glomerular filtrate. They produce substances which help in regulating blood pressure (renin–angiotensin system), formation of blood (erythropoietin), strengthening bones (active vitamin D/1,25-dihydroxyvitamin D) and protecting the kidneys from insults (prostaglandins and kinins) (*see* Chapter on Functions of the Kidney).

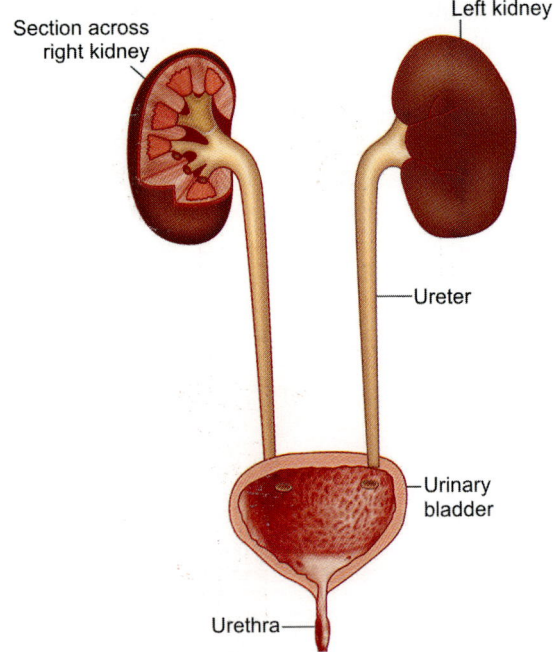

Fig. 1.1b: Urinary tract—female

Location

They are situated in the lumbar region (Fig. 1.2), one on either side of the vertebral column in the posterior abdominal wall. They are retroperitoneal in position, i.e. they are present behind the peritoneal cavity. The right kidney is at a slightly lower level compared to the left one because of the presence of liver on the right side between the kidney and the diaphragm.

Size and Shape

Each kidney measures approximately 11 cm × 6 cm × 3 cm, and is located between T_{11} and L_3 vertebral levels. It is bean shaped with concavity facing medially. The kidneys are tilted so that the upper poles lie closer to the midline, and the lower poles are directed away from the midline.

Hilum

The ureter emerges through the hilum, present at L_1 level. Other structures present at the hilum are the renal artery and the renal vein. Each kidney is supplied by the renal artery, a branch of abdominal aorta and is drained by the renal vein into the inferior vena cava.

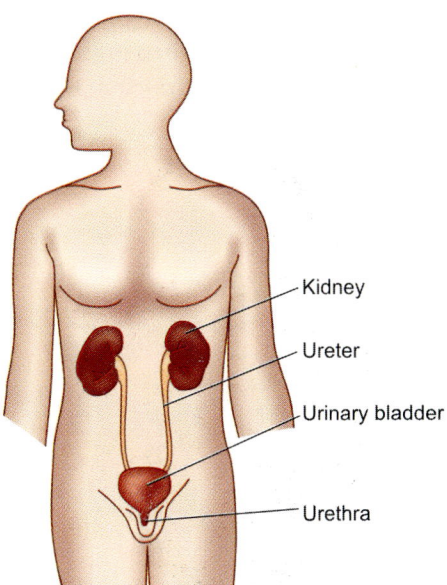

Fig. 1.2: Location of the kidneys

Coverings

Each kidney is surrounded by the following fascial coverings. They are important in supporting the kidney in position and protecting the kidneys from external injury. The coverings are from within outwards:

1. True capsule
2. Perirenal fat
3. Renal fascia
4. Pararenal fat

Loss of support by the fatty coverings, as in chronic debilitation, results in a clinical condition, called dropped kidney.

Internal Structure

Longitudinal section (Fig. 1.3) through the kidney shows that it consists of two parts— an outer cortex and an inner medulla. The cortex lies deep to the capsule and consists of nephrons. The medulla consists of 12–15 renal pyramids. The apical portions of the adjacent pyramids unite to form renal papillae. The renal papillae project into the minor calyces (calyx—singular; *kalyx means cup of a flower*). The collecting tubules pass through the pyramids and renal papillae and open into minor calyces. Minor calyces unite to form 3–4 major calyces, which in turn unite to form renal pelvis. Renal pelvis is the expanded upper portion of the ureter.

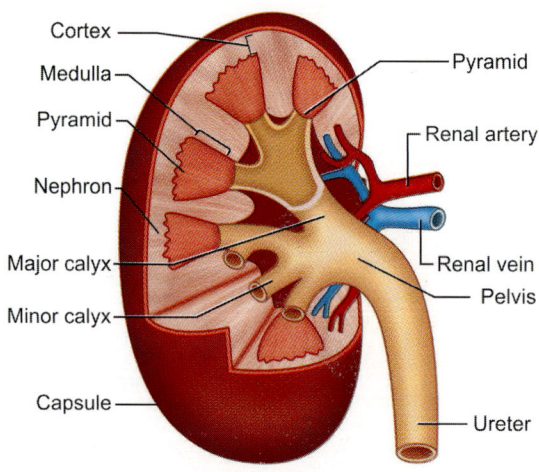

Fig. 1.3: Internal structure of the kidney

Nephron

Nephron is the structural and functional unit of the kidney. It consists of two parts, i.e. (1) renal corpuscle and (2) uriniferous tubule (Fig. 1.4).

Renal corpuscle is made up of two parts, namely the glomerulus and the Bowman's capsule. The glomerulus is a ball-like tuft of capillaries. The afferent arteriole enters and supplies blood to the capillary tuft and the efferent arteriole comes out draining the blood from it. The capillary tuft is surrounded by Bowman's capsule. The inner layer of the capsule is in contact with the glomerulus and is lined by highly specialized cells called podocytes. They play an important role in the filtration of urine.

Uriniferous tubule begins from the Bowman's capsule and consists of the following three parts:

1. Proximal convoluted tubule (PCT)
2. Loop of Henle
3. Distal convoluted tubule (DCT)

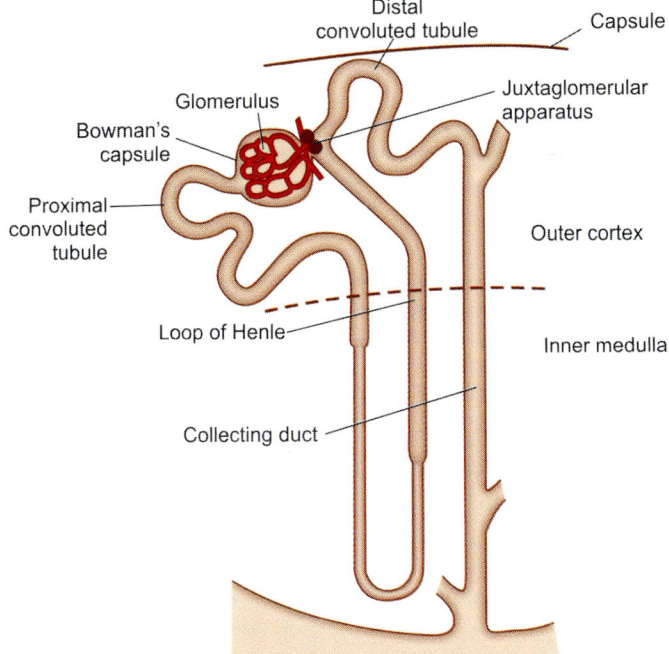

Fig. 1.4: Parts of the nephron

The PCTs are lined by tall columnar epithelium with a prominent brush border at the apical portions of the epithelial cells. They descend into the medulla and become continuous with the loop of Henle. The loop in turn has a descending limb and an ascending limb. The ascending limb re-enters the cortex to become continuous with the DCT. The DCTs are lined by short columnar cells without a brush border. The DCTs open into the collecting tubules which in turn open into the larger collecting ducts.

Juxtaglomerular Apparatus

This a specialized structure present where the glomerulus comes in contact with its own DCT. Here the cells of the DCT are modified and are called *macula densa*; and the smooth muscle cells of the afferent arteriole are modified to form the *juxtaglomerular (JG) cells*. These cells store renin as granules. The supporting cells between the macula densa and the JG cells are called *lacis cells*. The macula densa, JG cells and lacis cells together constitute the juxtaglomerular apparatus. The JG cells release renin under appropriate stimulus, and it plays an active role in regulation of blood pressure in the body.

Functionally, the kidney consists of two components:
1. Secretory part—constituted by the nephrons
2. Collecting part—constituted by the collecting tubules and ducts.

These two components develop separately from two different sources in the early embryonic life; and later get connected with each other.

Failure to establish connection between the two components results in various types of congenital polycystic kidney.

The kidneys are supplied by the renal arteries which are branches of abdominal aorta. The renal artery divides into lobar, interlobar, arcuate and interlobular arteries. Branches from the interlobular arteries are called afferent arterioles and each afferent arteriole supplies one glomerulus. The efferent arterioles, coming out of the glomeruli, form capillary plexus in the cortex and medulla. These capillary plexuses are drained by veins into the renal veins, which open into the inferior vena cava.

The renal nerves enter through a plexus (network) surrounding the arteries. There are no nerves transmitting pain sensation in the parenchyma. Only the renal capsule and renal pelvis are supplied by nerves transmitting pain sensation. Therefore, pain occurs only when the capsule is stretched or the renal pelvis distended or irritated.

URETER

The major calyces unite to form the renal pelvis which narrows down to continue as the ureter. The ureter is approximately 25 cm long. The upper half of the ureter lies in the abdomen and the lower half lies in the pelvis. It runs downwards along the anterior aspect of a muscle called psoas major. It then crosses the pelvic brim to enter the pelvic cavity. It initially runs down along the lateral wall of the pelvis. At the level of the ischial spine it turns forwards and medially to enter into the urinary bladder.

There are three normal constrictions in the ureter. These are:

1. At the pelviureteric junction (PUJ) (where the renal pelvis continues as the ureter, corresponds to level of lower pole of the kidney)
2. When the ureter crosses the pelvic brim.
3. When the ureter enters the bladder—vesicoureteric junction (VUJ).

These constrictions are the common sites of impaction by the ureteric stones.

- Narrowing of PUJ may be congenital and may lead to repeated infections or formation of stones in renal pelvis.
- Narrowing at the pelvic brim may cause impaction of stone here. During pregnancy, the ureter may be markedly distended to the level of pelvic brim due to the mechanical and hormonal factors.
- Impaction of stones at the VUJ is also common. Abnormalities at the VUJ may lead to reflux of urine from bladder into ureters—vesicoureteric reflux (VUR)

URINARY BLADDER

This is a hollow muscular organ which acts to store urine and discharge it periodically. When empty, it lies entirely in the pelvis. As the bladder fills up, it raises into the abdominal cavity pushing the peritoneum above it. A fully expanded bladder can reach the level of umbilicus.

An empty bladder resembles a three-sided pyramid, with its apex directed anteriorly towards the pubic symphysis. The base is directed posteriorly towards rectum in the males (Fig. 1.5) and is related to the seminal vesicles and the terminal part of vas deferens. The base is related to the vagina in the females (Fig. 1.6). The superior surface is related to the coils of small intestine and the sigmoid colon. The two inferolateral surfaces are related to the muscles in the lateral pelvic wall.

The lower end of the bladder is called the neck of the bladder. It corresponds to the internal urethral orifice and is surrounded by

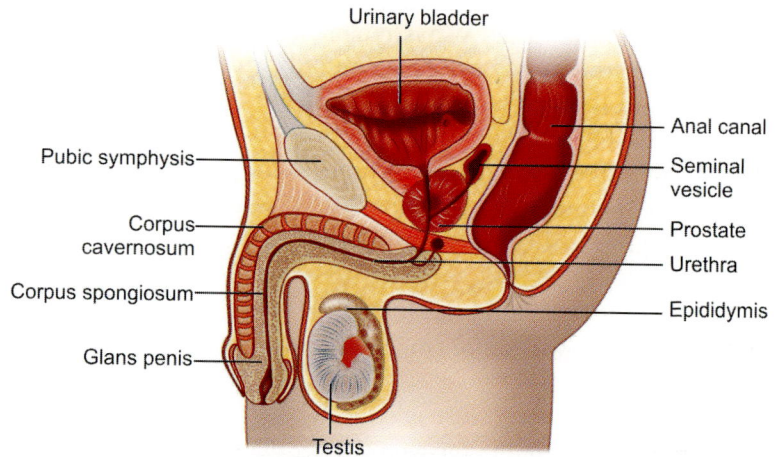

Fig. 1.5: Urinary bladder and parts of urethra in male

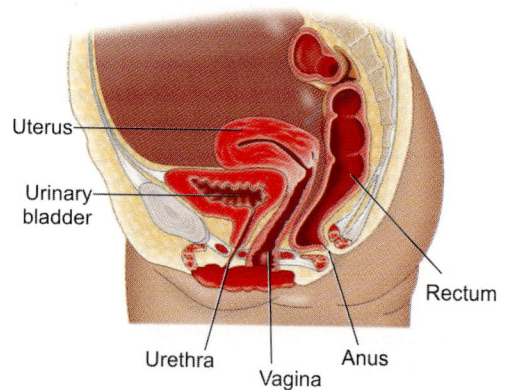

Fig. 1.6: Section of female pelvis showing urinary bladder and urethra

the internal urethral sphincter. The ureters open into the postero-lateral angles of the bladder, i.e. at the lateral angles of the base.

Trigone of the Bladder

The interior of the bladder presents a triangular area in the lower part of the posterior wall. This region is devoid of mucosal folds and is called the trigone of the bladder. It is bounded by the openings of the ureters at the upper and lateral angles, and the internal urethral orifice at the lower angle.

Detrusor Muscle

This is the muscle in the walls of the bladder. Parasympathetic stimulation is motor to the detrusor and inhibits the urethral sphincters; and thereby facilitates micturition. Sympathetic stimulation is inhibitory to detrusor and motor to the sphincters, thereby micturition does not take place.

The urinary bladder is supplied by branches from internal iliac arteries, and is drained by a venous plexus into internal iliac veins.

- Sometimes the anterior wall of urethra and the anterior abdominal wall fail to develop.
- In such cases, the trigone is exposed at the abdomen.
- This is a rare developmental anomaly, and is called ectopia vesicae.

MALE URETHRA

The male urethra is 20 cm long. It extends from the internal urethral orifice at the neck of the bladder to external urethral orifice at the tip of glans penis. It is divided into the following three parts (Fig. 1.7):

1. *Prostatic part*—3.5 cm, passes through the prostate gland. The ejaculatory ducts, that are formed by the union of the vas deferens and the seminal vesicle, open into this part of the urethra. Therefore, urethra forms the common passage for urine as well as the seminal fluid. This is the most dilatable part of urethra.

2. *Membranous part*—1.5 cm, the shortest, narrowest and the least dilatable of all the three parts. It is surrounded by the external urethral sphincter. It pierces the perineal membrane to enter into the root of the penis.

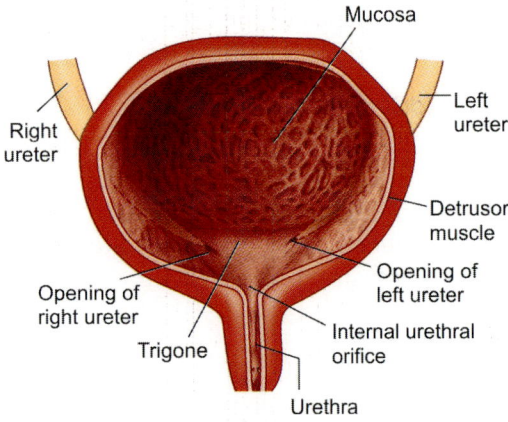

Fig. 1.7: Trigone of the bladder

3. *Penile part*—15 cm, the longest part of the urethra. It passes through the corpus spongiosum of the penis, and opens at the tip of the glans penis. The opening is called external urethral orifice/meatus.

- Sometimes the urethra opens on the ventral side of the penis. This condition is called hypospadias. Rarely, the urethra may open on the dorsum of the penis, and is known as epispadias.
- While inserting a catheter into the male urethra, it is important to remember that membranous part is the narrowest and the least dilatable part.

FEMALE URETHRA

The female urethra is very short (Fig. 1.6). It measures only 4 cm long. Developmentally, it corresponds to the prostatic part of urethra in the males. It runs along the anterior wall of vagina and opens in the pudendal cleft anterior to the vaginal opening.

- The short length of the urethra makes catheterization of urinary bladder easier in the female, but it makes the female urinary tract more prone to infections.
- Urinary tract infections (UTI) are more common in the females due to short urethra and ascent of infection.

2

Functions of the Kidneys and Mechanism of Urine Formation

Vikram Gowda, R Kasi Visweswaran

Kidneys are vital organs which play an important role in maintaining constant internal environment. They also perform the function of excretion of waste metabolites. The main functions are summarized below.

1. **Excretory function:** If the end products of metabolism accumulate in the body, it leads to imbalance in the functioning of cells and damage to tissues. So, they have to be excreted and this is performed by the kidneys. The main end products are urea (end product of protein metabolism), uric acid (nucleic acid metabolism), creatinine (skeletal muscle). Other substances like breakdown products of hemoglobin (bilirubin), metabolic end products of hormones, drugs, dyes, toxins or foreign substance are also excreted by the kidneys.

2. **Regulation of body fluid and osmolality:** Kidneys working together with cardiovascular system and central nervous system regulates the loss of water, sodium and other substances through kidneys. This is essential for maintenance of body fluid and osmolality. When a person is not getting sufficient water intake, the kidneys can reduce the urine volume and conserve water for the body. If the fluid intake is excessive, the kidneys help eliminate the excess water and maintain the normal water balance.

3. **Regulation of electrolytes:** Major inorganic ions such as sodium, potassium, calcium, chloride, bicarbonate, hydrogen and phosphate along with a few organic compounds are maintained within a normal range. This is done by regulating their excretion depending on the intake.

4. **Regulation of acid–base balance:** The pH of body fluids has to be maintained in a narrow range for normal functioning of the cells. Excess hydrogen ions or bicarbonate can alter the physiological activities. So, the acid–base balance has to be maintained in the blood and body fluid and is performed mainly by the kidneys.

5. **Endocrine functions:** The kidneys function like endocrine organ and liberate 5 important hormones.

a. *Renin:* Renin is an enzyme which activates renin–angiotensin–aldosterone axis which helps in long-term regulation of blood pressure. Thus, the kidneys play an important role in the long-term regulation of blood pressure. Kidney disease is an important cause of hypertension and hypertension can damage the kidneys also.

b. *Erythropoietin:* Erythropoietin is a protein secreted by the kidney and it acts on hematopoietic stem cells in bone marrow. Stimulation of erythropoiesis results in increased number of red blood corpuscles in circulation. Kidney diseases are associated with anemia which is related to deficiency of erythropoietin.

c. *Active vitamin D* (1, 25-dihydroxycholecalciferol): Kidneys secrete an enzyme 1α-hydroxylase which causes hydroxylation of 25-hydroxycholecalciferol to 1, 25-dihydroxycholecalciferol (calcitriol) which is the active form of vitamin D. This is an important hormone in regulation of calcium homeostasis. Children with renal disease develop rickets and adults may develop bone disease because of deficiency of active vitamin D.

d. *Prostaglandins*: Prostaglandins are produced in the kidney and they are involved in protecting the kidneys from damage due to transient hypotension and similar hemodynamic insults. This self-protection is called 'autoregulation'. Non-steroidal anti-inflammatory drugs (NSAIDs) suppress the activity of prostaglandins. So, this autoregulation is lost in patients taking NSAIDs and the kidneys can be damaged by even transient hypotension or other insults.

e. *Kinins* like bradykinins are the other hormones released in small quantity from kidneys which act as local vasodilators causing decrease in blood pressure and increase in tissue permeability in conditions of acute renal insult.

6. **Role in glucose metabolism:** Kidneys have an important role in glucose metabolism. About 50–60% of the insulin is degraded by the kidneys. In renal failure, this degradation may not occur. Therefore, the insulin may act for a longer duration and the diabetes may be well controlled with smaller doses of insulin. Gluconeogenesis means the production of glucose from non-carbohydrate substances like amino acids and fats (triglycerides). This function is also carried out by the kidneys. During prolonged fasting, the glucose level is maintained by conversion of triglycerides to glucose by the kidney. Thus, it helps in maintaining normal glucose concentration in plasma for proper functioning of vital organs like brain even during starvation.

Each kidney consists of approximately 1 million structural and functioning units called nephron. Each nephron has glomerulus which is surrounded by hollow capsule termed Bowman's capsule and space is formed within the capsule called Bowman's space (Fig. 2.1). This space continues as the tubular lumen. The

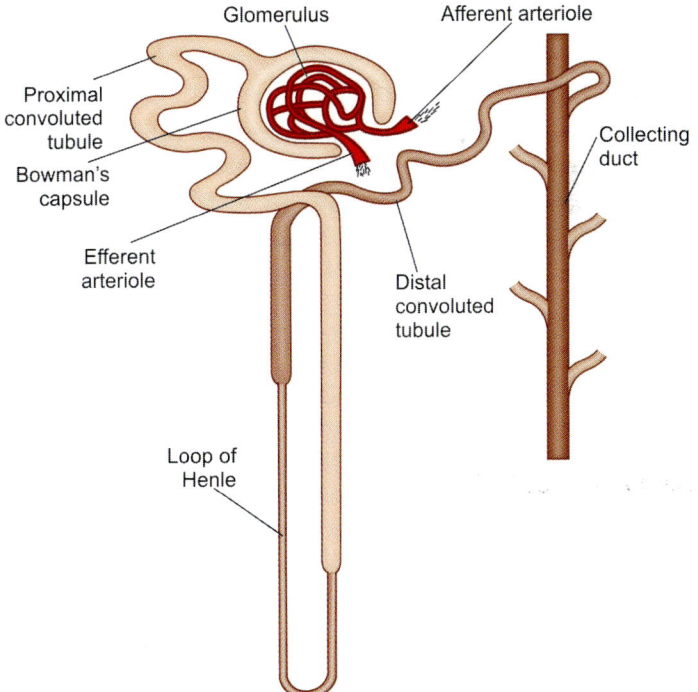

Fig. 2.1: Typical structure of nephron

tubule is about 5 cm long consists of a single layer of epithelial cells. But these cells are different in their structure and function in different parts of the nephron. The tubule is divided into proximal tubule, loop of Henle, distal tubule and collecting duct. The kidneys are supplied with blood from the aorta through renal arteries— usually one on each side which divide inside the kidney and supply the glomerulus. The branch of the renal artery entering the glomerulus is called afferent arteriole. In the glomerulus, it divides into small capillaries and re-group to form the efferent arteriole which subsequently forms a network of capillaries around the tubule. The venous system is formed from these capillaries and the blood is returned through the renal veins into the inferior vena cava.

MECHANISM OF URINE FORMATION

Urine formation involves three major processes:

1. Filtration by the glomeruli,
2. Tubular reabsorption and
3. Tubular secretion in the renal tubules.

In the nephron, the three processes mentioned above occur in a coordinated manner to form urine.

GLOMERULAR FILTRATION

The glomerulus acts as a filter and forms an ultrafiltrate from blood. All substances dissolved in plasma and small molecular weight substances are filtered here. The rate at which the glomerulus filters is called *glomerular filtration rate (GFR)*. In a healthy adult, GFR averages about 125 ml/min, i.e. 180 L/day. From this filtrate, nearly 178–179 L is reabsorbed by the tubule leaving about 1–2 L of urine formed daily. Thus, nearly 99% or more of the filtrate is normally reabsorbed. The factors controlling GFR include size of the capillary bed, the permeability of the capillaries, and the hydrostatic and osmotic pressure gradients across the capillary wall.

Capillary Permeability

The glomerular capillary wall, together with the basement membrane and epithelial cell functions as a filter. The sialoproteins in the glomerular capillary wall provide negative charge. Therefore, negatively charged substances in blood, like albumin with a molecular diameter of 7 nm, are not filtered by the glomerulus. In diseases of the glomerulus, the negative charge is lost and there is usually increased filtration and excretion of albumin in urine.

Filtration of substances with positive charge (cationic substances) is greater than that of neutral substances.

Filtration Surface Area

The mesangial cells can alter the effective area in the glomerular capillary for filtration. When the mesangium contracts, there is a reduction in the area available for filtration decrease in filtration and vice versa.

Hydrostatic and Oncotic Pressures

The pressure in the glomerular capillaries is very high when compared to other systemic capillaries. This is because of the short length of arterioles and distance between the aorta and glomerular capillaries compared to the capillaries in the finger tip. The efferent arterioles have a relatively higher resistance because of short and decreased diameter than afferent arteriole. The pressure in the glomerular capillary (capillary hydrostatic pressure) mainly controls the filtration. The glomerular filtration rate (GFR) is approximately 125 ml/min. Changes in the GFR can occur due to decreased filtration permeability, damage of the endothelial lining or alteration of hydrostatic pressure in capillaries.

Tubular Reabsorption

This process called tubular reabsorption is selective and occurs from the lumen of the tubule to the peritubular capillaries through the cell (transepithelial) or through the space between the cells (paracellular route). It begins as soon as the filtrate enters the proximal tubules. In the transcellular route, transported substances move through the luminal membrane, the cytosol, and the basolateral membrane of the tubule cell and then the endothelium of the peritubular capillaries. Movement of substances in the paracellular route between the tubule cells is limited because these cells are connected by tight junctions. In the proximal nephron, these tight junctions are "leaky" and allow some ions (Ca^{2+}, Mg^{2+}, K^+, and Na^+) through the paracellular route.

All organic nutrients such as glucose and amino acids are completely reabsorbed to maintain or restore normal plasma concentrations. On the other hand, the reabsorption of water and many ions is continuously regulated and adjusted in response to hormonal signals. Depending on the substances transported, the reabsorption process may be passive (no ATP required) or active (ATP required).

SODIUM REABSORPTION

Sodium ions are freely filtered from the blood and reach the tubular fluid (Fig. 2.2). From here, it is reabsorbed actively through the

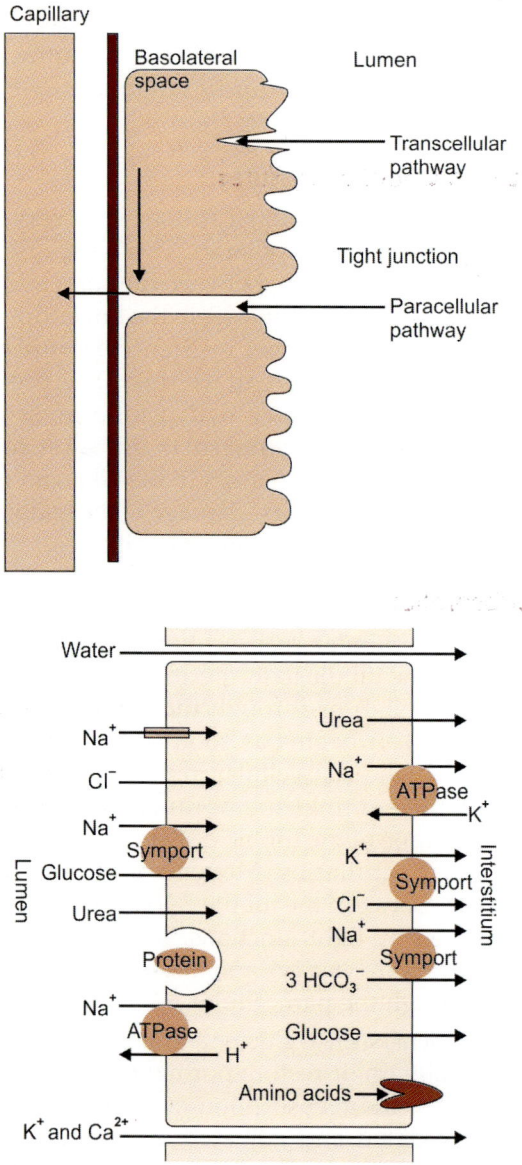

Fig. 2.2: Transport of substances across epithelium in kidney tubules

transcellular route. Various segments of the nephron are involved in sodium reabsorption which is an active process utilizing energy. Sodium reabsorption utilizes about 80% of the energy used for active transport in the kidney. In general, two basic processes that promote active Na reabsorption occur in each tubule segment. First, Na enters the tubular cell through the luminal membrane. From the cell, it is transported to the peritubular space by primary active transport via Na^+, K^+-ATPase pump in the basolateral membrane. From there, Na moves along with water into adjacent peritubular capillaries. About 60–70% is reabsorbed in the proximal tubule together with identical percentage of water (iso-osmotic reabsorption). In the thick ascending limb of the loop of Henle, about 25% of the water is reabsorbed together with potassium and chloride. In the distal tubule, about 7–9% reabsorption occurs in exchange for potassium and this is controlled by the adrenal hormone aldostrerone. Nearly 99% of filtered sodium is reabsorbed and about 1% is excreted in the urine. In conditions of dehydration, sodium is reabsorbed almost completely and the urinary sodium is lower than 1%. If the tubule is damaged, urinary sodium may be higher than 2%. When the patient is administered diuretics, the urinary sodium may be high. Thus, urinary sodium can be used as a test to find if tubules are functioning normally (if the patient has not been given diuretic).

REABSORPTION OF NUTRIENTS, WATER, AND IONS

The reabsorption of Na^+ by primary active transport is the force which enables the reabsorption of substances like water, glucose, amino acids, lactate, and vitamins. In all these cases, substances are transported across the membrane as cotransport (symport) or countertransport (antiport) with another solute. There is a maximum capacity for transport of a substance across a membrane [transport maximum (Tm)]. The Tm (mg/min) reflects the number of transport proteins in the renal tubules available to transport each particular substance. For substances such as glucose that need to be reabsorbed completely from lumen, there are numerous transporters. Therefore, Tm values are high. For substances which have to be excreted or of less significance to body, there may be a few or no transporters. When the transporters are saturated by the substrates, the excess substrates in lumen are excreted in urine. For example, in uncontrolled diabetes, when plasma glucose exceeds 180 mg/dl, the glucose Tm is exceeded and the unabsorbed glucose is lost in the urine. Here, the tubule is functioning normally. In a condition called renal glycosuria, there is a tubular abnormality by which the Tm for glucose is lower than normal and so the patient may have sugar in urine even though the blood sugar is within the normal range.

Passive tubular reabsorption occurs by osmosis, diffusion, and facilitated diffusion. Substances move down their electrochemical gradients without need for energy (use of ATP). This occurs due to the osmotic gradient created by sodium and other solutes. Water moves by osmosis through water channels called aquaporin channels that form water channels across cell membranes. In proximal tubules, water reabsorption occurs constantly and aquaporin channels are constantly present in the cell wall and the reabsorption is constant (obligatory water reabsorption). The presence or absence of aquaporin in the collecting is regulated by antidiuretic hormone (ADH).

The PCT reabsorbs all of the glucose, lactate, and amino acids in the glomerular filtrate together with filtrate and 65–70% of the Na^+ and water. About 80% of the filtered bicarbonate (HCO_3^-), uric acid, 60% of the Cl, about 55% of the K^+ and 50% of urea are reabsorbed in PCT. However, urea and uric acid are secreted in the distal tubule.

In the loop of Henle, the permeability of the tubule epithelium is entirely different. Here, water reabsorption occurs in the descending limb of the loop of Henle but not the ascending limb. The water leaves the descending (but not the ascending) limb of Henle's loop, and the solutes the opposite occurs. $Na^+–K^+–2Cl^-$ symport pump is responsible for active reabsorption of sodium, potassium and chloride in the luminal surface in the thick portion of the ascending limb. The thick ascending limb also has $Na^+–H^+$ antiport pumps.

By the time the DCT is reached, only about 10% of the originally filtered NaCl and 25% of the water remain in the tubule. Most reabsorption from this point depends on the body's needs at the time and is regulated by hormones mainly aldosterone for Na^+, ADH for water, and PTH for Ca^{2+}. If necessary, nearly all of the water and Na^+ reaching these regions can be reabsorbed.

In the absence of antidiuretic hormone (ADH), the collecting ducts are relatively impermeable to water and more volume of urine is formed. If ADH is present, reabsorption of more water occurs and the urine volume is reduced. Aldosterone helps in reabsorption of the remaining Na^+. Aldosterone is released from the adrenal cortex in response to decreased blood volume, blood pressure, extracellular Na^+ concentration (hyponatremia), or high extracellular K^+ concentration (hyperkalemia). Hyperkalemia directly stimulates the adrenal cortex to secrete aldosterone. Other conditions stimulate the renin-angiotensin mechanism, which in turn releases aldosterone. Aldosterone causes increased reabsorption of the Na^+ in the DCT segment in exchange for K^+ which is secreted into the tubule. If aldosterone is absent, less Na^+ is reabsorbed by these segments, resulting in abnormal urinary losses of Na^+. Aldosterone is important in maintaining blood volume and blood pressure and excess aldosterone causes sodium retention and hypokalemia.

In contrast to aldosterone, atrial natriuretic peptide (ANP), released by cardiac atria cells when blood volume or blood pressure is elevated, reduces blood Na^+, thereby decreasing blood volume and blood pressure. ANP also directly inhibits Na^+ reabsorption at the collecting ducts.

TUBULAR SECRETION

The tubules are able to excrete unwanted substances from the body by not reabsorbing them along the tubule (e.g. creatinine). By tubular secretion, it adds certain unwanted solutes to the urine and eliminates them from the body (e.g. H^+, K^+, NH_4^+, and certain organic acids). They either move into the filtrate from the peritubular capillaries through the tubule cells or are synthesized in the tubule cells and secreted. As a result, the urine eventually excreted contains both filtered and secreted substances.

One of the important functions of tubular secretion is constant maintenance of body fluid and pH which is done by concentrating the tubular fluid and excreting H^+ ions and generating HCO_3. When blood pH tends to reduce, the renal tubule cells actively secrete more H^+ into the filtrate and retain and generate more HCO_3^-. As a result, the blood pH rises and the urine drains off the excess H^+. Conversely, when blood pH tends to increase, Cl reabsorbed instead of HCO_3^- which is allowed to be excreted.

Drugs and metabolites that are tightly bound to plasma proteins have to be excreted. Because plasma proteins are not filtered, the substances bound to them are not filtered and so must be secreted into the lumen through the tubule. Tubular secretion is also essential for excretion of end products like urea and uric acid that have been reabsorbed.

We conclude that glomerulus is the primary site where filtration of the plasma occurs selectively for substances of cationic followed by neutral and least for anions based on their molecular size. The filtered fluid is iso-osmotic to the plasma, PCT is the primary site where we noticed the maximum reabsorption of substrates, that is about 60% of all substances except glucose which is 100% reabsorbed in PCT and secretion of substances which are to be excreted and acidification of urine is done simultaneously as the filtrate reaches loop of Henle, where descending limb is permeable only to water and ascending limb permeable only to electrolytes. Reabsorption occurs along with concentration of urine majorly by countercurrent mechanism and in this site nearly 10% of the substrates are reabsorbed and filtrate reaching DCT and collecting duct remaining 5% of the substrates are reabsorbed mainly in the presence of hormones (ADH and aldosterone) along with secretion of substances and acidification of filtrate which is passed down as urine.

3

Development and Development Anomalies of Urinary Tract

R Hema, John Joseph

The cells in the embryo differentiate into ectoderm, mesoderm and endoderm. The kidney develops from the mesoderm. There are three successive phases in the development of the kidney—called pronephros, mesonephros and metanephros. The pronephros is the first to develop and consists of tube-like structures in the part of the embryo which forms the neck of the fetus. It disappears completely as the embryo grows. The mesonephros arises from the mesoderm in the thoracic region of the embryo. The mesonephros is also a set of tube-like structures which unite to form a duct called mesonephric duct or Wolffian duct. The mesonephric duct ends in the cloaca which is the urogenital sinus. It is here that the gastrointestinal and urinary tract opens. The cloaca further develops as the urinary bladder and the rectum. The kidney develops from metanephros in the pelvic region. During the 5th week of gestation, a projection like a diverticulum develops from the mesonephric duct near the opening of this duct into the cloaca. This projection is called the ureteric bud. The bud grows into the metanephros, undergoes a series of branching and ultimately develops to form the collecting duct, calyces, renal pelvis and ureter. The portion of undifferentiated intermediate mesoderm (metanephros) which is in contact with the branching ureteric bud, is known as metanepheric blastema (Fig. 3.1). The ureteric bud induces the formation of the tubules in this metanephric blastema. The vascular endothelial cells at the tips of renal tubules differentiate into cells of the glomerulus. Thus a nephron unit is formed. As the renal tubules grow, they join with collecting duct system resulting in continuity of flow. The development of kidneys is complete by 32–36 weeks of intrauterine life. However, the renal functions

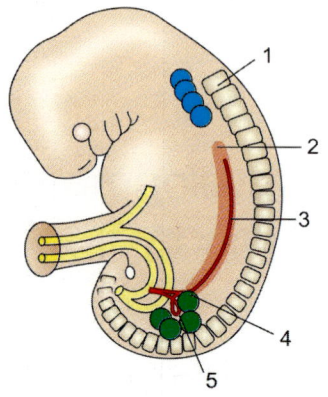

1. Region of development of pronephros (blue)
2. Mesonephros—orange
3. Mesonephric duct (wolffian duct)—red
4. Metanephric blastema (develops into kidney)—green
5. Ureteric bud (develops into collecting system)—red (branch of mesonephric duct)

Fig. 3.1: Embryo and the position of pronephros, mesonephros and metanephros

improve over the first 2 years and the maturity continues to develop ever after birth.

MIGRATION OF THE KIDNEY

The metanephros develops into the kidney in the pelvic cavity and ascends subsequently to its normal position in the lumbar region. This occurs due to the lengthwise growth and straightening of the fetus. As the kidney ascends, it acquires blood supply from the adjacent aorta. The vessels that supply the kidney in the pelvic position degenerate and only the renal arteries which arise from the abdominal aorta persist when fully developed.

CONGENITAL ANOMALIES OF KIDNEYS AND URETERS

Congenital abnormalities of the urinary system are common and may be seen in 3–4% of neonates. Most abnormalities can be diagnosed by antenatal sonography. The common abnormalities include those due to abnormal position, rotation and number of kidneys. Other abnormalities include anomalies in the ureter, vesicoureteric junction or urinary bladder.

Renal Agenesis

Agenesis of the kidneys may be seen in 1 in 1000 live-births. It is more common on the left side. Males are more affected than females and may be associated with left-sided testicular agenesis. If unilateral, the patients are usually asymptomatic. Bilateral agenesis is associated with severe oligohydramnios, peculiar facial appearance called 'Potter' facies and is incompatible with life. Such fetus are often stillborn.

Ectopic Kidneys

Ectopic kidney means that the kidney is not in its normal position in the loin. One or both kidneys can be affected. They may be present in any position along the line of the normal ascent of the kidney. Pelvic kidneys are the commonest and they get blood vessels from adjacent aorta (Fig. 3.2). Thoracic kidneys are very rare. In thoracic kidney, one or both kidneys may be in the thorax. Sometimes, both kidneys may be on the same side. This is called crossed renal ectopia. The 2 kidneys may be entirely separate and on the right or left side or may be fused with one another. In this condition, the ureters join the bladder on either side.

Horseshoe Kidneys

Horseshoe kidney results due to connection between the lower pole of both kidneys. This connection may consist of functioning renal tissue or even fibrous band. This connection is called the isthmus. Because of the presence of the isthmus, the kidney is unable to ascend because the inferior mesenteric artery from the aorta will block the ascent and prevent kidney from reaching its

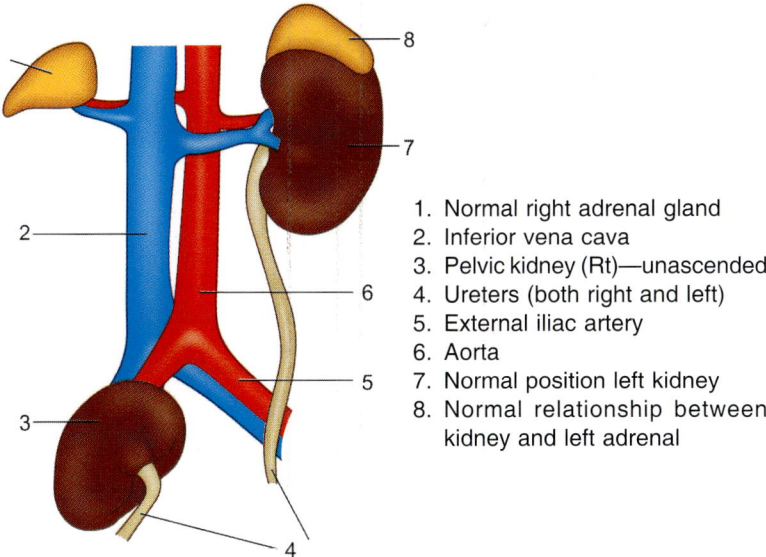

1. Normal right adrenal gland
2. Inferior vena cava
3. Pelvic kidney (Rt)—unascended
4. Ureters (both right and left)
5. External iliac artery
6. Aorta
7. Normal position left kidney
8. Normal relationship between kidney and left adrenal

Fig. 3.2: Showing (unascended) pelvic kidney

normal position in the lumbar region. The large single U-shaped kidney lies in the pubic region and its lower poles are fused (Fig. 3.3). Such kidneys are prone to nephrolithiasis, hypertension, infection, obstruction or tumors. Whenever the kidneys are prevented from ascending to their normal position, the rotation may not be complete and such malpositioned kidneys are also malrotated. Rotation anomalies result in abnormal position of hilum of the kidney. In normal kidney, the hilum faces medially. The hilum of the kidney with above anomaly may face anteriorly, laterally or even posteriorly.

DUPLICATION OF URINARY TRACT

Duplication of the collecting system may result from abnormal or incomplete division of the ureteric bud resulting in complete or partial double ureters. In complete duplication, there may be 2 collecting systems and ureters draining separately into the bladder on the same side. Sometimes the anomaly can be bifid pelvis or ureter draining one kidney. Renal duplication means that there are 2 kidneys with one ureter for each kidney which opens into the same side in the bladder. Note that in renal duplication the 2 ureters join the bladder on the same side, whereas in crossed ectopia, they join the bladder on either side. Formation of more

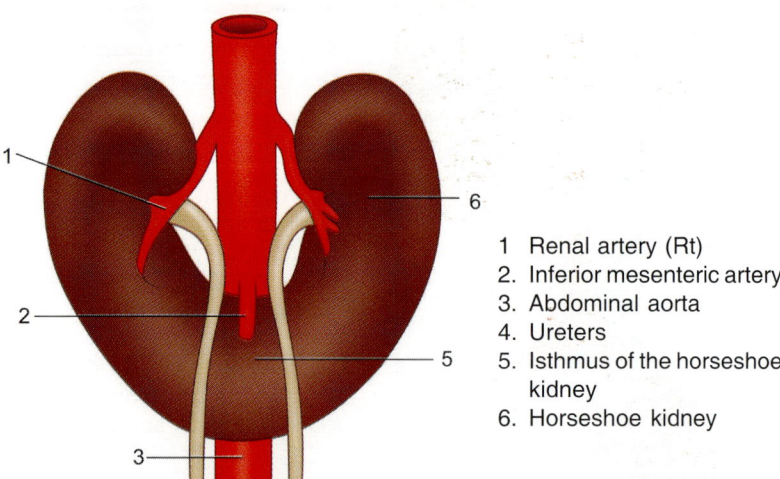

1 Renal artery (Rt)
2. Inferior mesenteric artery
3. Abdominal aorta
4. Ureters
5. Isthmus of the horseshoe kidney
6. Horseshoe kidney

Fig. 3.3: Horseshoe kidney—the ascent of the kidney is blocked by inferior mesenteric artery

than one ureteric bud on the same sides results in supernumerary kidney.

Ectopic Ureter

Under normal conditions, the ureter opens in the trigone of the bladder. Here, the ureter travels through an oblique tunnel through the muscle and submucosal area of the bladder wall. The arrangement of the muscular fibres here and the intramural tunnel prevents the urine from the bladder going into the ureter during micturition. If the ureter opens anywhere other than the trigone of the bladder, it may not be able to prevent the backflow of urine from the bladder to ureter. This backflow during micturition is called vesicoureteral reflux (VUR). When the ectopic ureteric opening lies in bladder neck, urethra or vagina, it may result in dribbling of urine (urinary incontinence).

Ureterocele

In this condition, there is dilatation of the end of the ureter that projects into the bladder and may present with recurrent urinary tract infection during childhood.

CYSTIC DISEASES OF THE KIDNEYS

Cysts in the kidney can be congenital or acquired, single or multiple, unilateral or bilateral, simple or complicated and genetically transmitted or otherwise. (Please see the chapter on cysts of the kidney.)

Megaureters and VUR

Megaureters are abnormally dilated ureters and result from either obstruction (ureterocels or primary obstructing megaureter) or following vesicoureteral reflux (VUR). VUR is a very common anomaly in children where there is partial flow of urine in the reverse direction from urinary bladder into the ureter at rest or during micturition. Such patients are prone to urinary tract infection. Infected urine passes into the kidneys through the ureter if there is VUR and this results in renal infection (pyelonephritis) leading to kidney damage and renal scars (reflux nephropathy).

As explained earlier, VUR results from the absence of submucosal tunnel of ureter before the ureter opens into the bladder. Depending on the severity, reflux is graded into grade 1 to 5. Diagnosis is confirmed by micturiting cystourethrography (MCU), identifying renal scars and assessing renal functions. Treatment depends on the severity of the reflux. Grades 1 and 2 are milder forms of reflux and are usually managed medically. Grades 4 and 5 are severe forms and may need surgical correction. Surgical reimplantation into the bladder to prevent reflux (ureteric reimplantation or ureteroneocystostomy) or injection of 'teflon' near the ureteric opening in the bladder are the surgical options.

Pelviureteric Junction Obstruction (PUJ Obstruction)

Obstruction or narrowing of the junction between the renal pelvis and beginning of the ureter is a common congenital anomaly. This may result in enlargement of the renal pelvis, calyces and kidney (hydronephrosis). The causes may be due to factors outside the wall (extraparietal), in the wall of the ureter (parietal), or inside the lumen (intraparietal). Abnormal artery to the lower pole of the kidney is the most common extraparietal cause. Parietal causes due to abnormal distribution of muscular and collagen fibres at PUJ are more common.

Children with this abnormality present with recurrent abdominal pain, UTI, renal swelling (mass) or hematuria. Diagnosis is made by USG which measures the anteroposterior diameter of renal pelvis at the renal hilum. Any measurement above 20 mm is significant. Other investigations are DTPA renogram and intravenous urogram.

Surgical correction is by excising the PUJ and constructing a dependent ureteropelvic anastomosis (pyeloplasty).

4

Kidney Diseases in Infants and Children

Leni Kumar Joseph, Sushama Bai

Kidney diseases are common in children. Often the symptoms are mild and the diagnosis is delayed. Kidney disease should be suspected in children if there is a history of kidney disease in other members of the family. The usual presenting features of kidney diseases in children are:

1. **Edema:** Puffiness of eyelids, face, ankles, legs and later, swelling of the body.
2. **Hematuria:** Blood in urine (red/coffee-coloured urine), RBCs on microscopy.
3. **Oliguria:** Urine volume <0.5 ml/kg body weight/hour in children or anuria.
4. **Dysuria/abdominal pain:** Pain (crying) on passing urine.
5. **Frequency of micturition:** Passing urine ≥8 times per day.
6. **Polyuria:** Increased urine volume >4 ml/kg body weight/ hour.
7. **Abnormalities in micturition:** Dribbling of urine, incontenance (lack of control of urination), nocturnal enuresis.
8. **Hypertension:** BP >95th percentile of normal for age ± complications.
9. Poor physical growth especially with bony deformities and/or anemia.
10. Abnormalities on investigations (urine, blood or imaging studies).

Most of the disorders that occur in adults can occur in children also. Some disorders are more common in children. Only the important features in children are discussed in this chapter. Development of the kidneys and urinary system and abnormalities in development are discussed in a separate chapter. Common disorders seen in children are:

1. Nephrotic syndrome
2. Acute nephritis/acute glomerulonephritis
3. Acute kidney injury/A/c renal failure
4. Chronic kidney disease/ C/c renal failure
5. Urinary tract infection
6. Renal tubular disorders
7. Abnormalities in micturition and nocturnal enuresis
8. Hypertension due to renal/renovascular causes.

    (Please see the independent chapters for full description)

NEPHROTIC SYNDROME (NS)

Nephrotic syndrome is defined as excretion of large amounts of protein in urine (≥2 gm/m^2 body surface area) often accompanied by edema, low serum albumin (hypoalbuminemia < 3.5 g/dl) and hypercholesterolemia (>250 mg/dl). The causes in children are usually due to primary glomerular disease and very rarely secondary to systemic diseases (e.g. SLE)/infections (like hepatitis B, malaria, HIV). If NS occurs in infants <1 year, it is mostly congenital NS. In children in the age group of 2–8 years, the condition is predominantly minimal change nephrotic syndrome (MCNS). This is the commonest form of NS in children. In minimal change MCNS if kidney biopsy is done, it shows no significant changes on light microscopy. Even in adolescents, MCNS is common but other primary glomerulopathies may also occur.

   Children with congenital NS have structural defects of the glomerular capillary filter but in most childhood NS there is damage to the glomerular basement membrane which is mediated by the immune system. Because of the damage, there is protein leak into the urine, loss of protein from the body, low serum albumin, low colloid osmotic pressure of blood, fluid leak from blood to extracellular fluid compartment, edema, lower blood volume, salt and water retention by the kidney and worsening of edema (Fig. 4.1). The attempt of the liver to increase protein synthesis results in more synthesis of lipids.

   The onset is gradual and the mother notices puffiness of the face on waking up from sleep which progresses to pedal edema. In later stages, there may be gross edema with edema of genitals, ascites and pleural effusion. This is called anasarca. Some children present

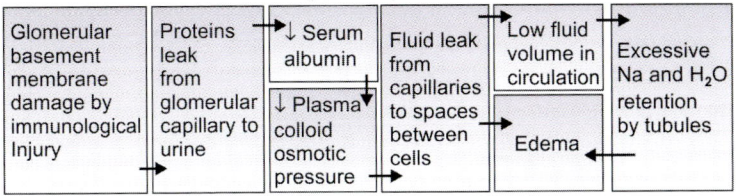

| Glomerular basement membrane damage by immunological Injury | Proteins leak from glomerular capillary to urine | ↓ Serum albumin ↓ Plasma colloid osmotic pressure | Fluid leak from capillaries to spaces between cells | Low fluid volume in circulation Edema | Excessive Na and H₂O retention by tubules |

Fig. 4.1: Edema formation in nephrotic syndrome

with symptoms due to complications like peritonitis or thrombosis. Investigations are similar to adults. In children, spot urine protein –creatinine ratio is preferred to 24-hour urine protein. Kidney biopsy is generally not indicated in typical childhood NS. The indications for biopsy in children include occurrence before 1 year or after 12 years of age, presence of atypical features like hematuria, hypertension or renal failure. In steroid dependant NS, biopsy is often done before starting calcinurin inhibitors like cyclosporine or Tacrolimus. Screening for hidden infections like tuberculosis and screening for viruses like hepatitis B and C should be done before starting treatment. Medications used for NS will suppress immunity and could cause serious flare up of hidden infections.

The line of treatment is immunosuppression by steroids. Prednisolone in doses of 60 mg/m² body surface area daily for 4–6 weeks (approximately 2 mg/kg body wt) and then two-thirds the dose on alternate days for 4–6 weeks. Depending on the response, the dosage is tapered and stopped by 3 months. The diet advised should contain adequate protein and low fat intake. The fluid intake is regulated depending on the severity of edema and volume of urine output. Salt restriction is necessary for patients who are edematous. Diuretics and albumin infusions are used to control anasarca.

The prognosis is generally good. Depending on the response, they can be classified as:

a. *Steroid-sensitive NS:* Children respond with no protein in urine
b. *Remission:* Patient continues to remain well with no proteinuria
c. *Lasting remission:* Remains in remission for many years.
d. *Relapse:* When patient responds and proteinuria reappears (> ++)

e. *Steroid dependant NS:* When relapse occurs two times while steroid dose is reduced or within 2–4 weeks of stopping treatment.

f. *Frequently relapsing NS:* Relapse occurs more than 2 times in 6 months or >3 times a year.

g. *Infrequently relapsing NS:* Frequency of relapse <2 times a year.

h. *Steroid resistant NS:* Continues to have proteinuria after 4 weeks of daily dose. These children may progress to renal failure later.

Renal biopsy is done for frequently relapsing, steroid dependant and steroid resistant nephrotic syndromes before using more powerful immunosuppressive drugs.

ACUTE NEPHRITIS, ACUTE GLOMERULONEPHRITIS (AGN)

Acute nephritic syndrome consists of sudden onset of hematuria, oliguria, hypertension and usually moderate proteinuria. In childhood, it occurs as a manifestation of post-infectious acute glomerulonephritis (PSAGN) and follows streptococcal throat/skin infection. Rarely, other bacterial, viral infections, infective endocarditis, vasculitides and systemic disorders may involve kidneys and present as AGN. Simplified pathogenesis is shown in Fig. 4.2. Streptococcal/other antigens stimulate formation of antibodies in the body. The antibody binds to the antigens; the complexes thus formed get deposited in the glomeruli, attract inflammatory cells which release inflammatory mediators (cytokines) setting up a chain reaction of capillary damage, GFR reduction and salt and water retention.

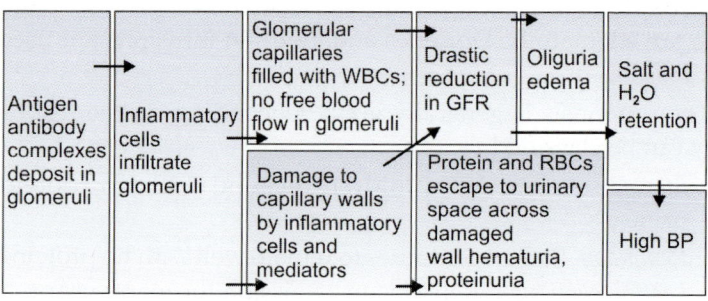

Fig. 4.2: How inflammation leads to clinical manifestations of AGN-simplified diagram

Clinical features and presentation may vary from subclinical to typical symptoms and signs of acute nephritis (red or cola coloured urine, edema, oliguria or anuria, hypertension or its complications, hypertensive encephalopathy, seizure, altered consciousness, acute pulmonary edema or cardiac failure). Urinalysis will show protein, RBCs, WBCs and casts. Serum creatinine and blood urea may be elevated or normal. Electrolytes (especially K^+) should be monitored. Special tests like serum complement (C_3, C_4), ANA, antistreptolysin O (ASO) are useful. PSAGN is self-limiting and treatment is supportive. Fluid intake is restricted to the previous day's output volume + the estimated insensible fluid loss from the body (400–600 ml/m^2 body surface area). Salt and potassium intake are restricted. For control of hypertension and fluid retention, diuretics and antihypertensives are given, a course of antibiotics is advised only if active skin or throat infection is present.

Outcome of AGN depends on the underlying cause. PSAGN almost always recover without significant residual kidney damage and does not recur. Hypertension and edema subside in 2–3 weeks and gross hematuria within ~4 weeks but urine microscopy may show RBCs for 6–12 months. The children are followed up periodically.

URINARY TRACT INFECTION (UTI) IN CHILDREN

Infection of the urinary tract is the growth of a significant number of organisms of a single species in the urine, in the presence of symptoms/significant pyuria. The commonly used terms and their meanings are explained in Table 4.1. UTI is usually caused by bacteria in the patient's own gut, usually *E. coli.* Other organisms like Klebsiella, Proteus and other Gram-negative bacilli may be seen in complicated UTIs.

Table 4.1: Common terms and their meanings

Significant bacteriuria	>50,000 colonies/ml of single species grown in midstream clean catch sample
Significant pyuria	>5 pus cells (WBCs) per high power field in a centrifuged sample
Asymptomatic bacteriuria	Significant bacteriuria in the absence of pyuria/symptoms of UTI
Sterile pyuria	Significant pyuria on microscopy but no significant bacterial growth in culture

Urine and urinary tract are normally maintained sterile because of the normal epithelial lining (urothelium) and by constant flushing out of organisms by regular flow of urine. Any stagnation of urine in the bladder—due to anatomical obstruction/incomplete emptying/infrequent voiding/back-leak into ureters (VU reflux) will result in bacteria attaching to the urothelium multiplying. Thus, urothelial damage from trauma, surgery, instrumentation or stones enables bacteria to adhere firmly to the mucosa. Gram-negative bacilli having fimbriae that can adhere strongly to mucosa so that they are not flushed out. They ascend to the upper tract (ureters and kidneys) in presence of reflux and cause pyelonephritis (infection of kidney and collecting system) or sepsis.

Clinical features depend on age and general condition of child and severity of infection.

Simple UTI affecting lower urinary tract may be associated with low grade fever, frequency of micturition, urgency, pain, straining and crying while passing urine and absence of findings of complicated UTI. In infection of upper urinary tract, the child could have all the symptoms experienced by the adult (high fever, loin pain, body ache, and loin tenderness). Sometimes they may have only vomiting.

Urine microscopy and culture are necessary to confirm the diagnosis. Because of the difficulty in getting a clean catch, mid-stream urine sample for culture without external contamination, suprapubic aspiration of the sample from the bladder is taken for culture. Blood counts and blood culture, serum creatinine and electrolytes are needed in complicated UTIs. About 30% of children with UTIs may have underlying anatomical defects (causing urinary obstruction/backflow (reflux)/stagnation). So, ultrasound scan of abdomen will help to diagnose most of these. Further imaging methods are needed as follows:

a. Age <1 year   USG, MCU, DMSA scan.
b. Age 1–5 years   USG, DMSA scan—if abnormal MCU.
c. Age >5 years   USG only—if abnormal, MCU, DMSA scan

Ultrasonogram (USG) shows urine/pus collection, stones, mass in kidney.

Micturating cystourethrogram (MCU) also called voiding cystourethrogram (VCUG) can show obstruction, reflux of urine from bladder to ureter during voiding.

DMSA scan (DMSA = Tc 99 dimercaptosuccinic acid radioisotope renogram) shows scars in the kidney due to pyelonephritis.

Treatment is general and specific. Adequate fluid intake and regular voiding is essential. Bowel-bladder dysfunction (infrequent voiding and/or constipation) is managed with diet high fluid and fibre intake, timed voiding and bowel-bladder training. Simple UTIs may be treated with oral antibiotics but complicated UTIs require injections till child tolerates oral medications. Antibiotics are given as per culture sensitivity report for 10–14 days even though the symptoms may subside after 3–4 days. Those with reflux are taught double voiding and may be given long-term antibiotic chemoprophylaxis. Severe reflux/obstructions will need surgical correction. Pyelonephritis with/without reflux may lead to renal scarring resulting in hypertension and chronic kidney disease in later life.

NOCTURNAL ENURESIS (NE)

Usually a child is able to control micturition and not pass urine in bed during sleep (bed wetting) after the age of 5 years. Primary NE is a condition in which the child had never attained night-time bladder control (if a child >5 years old passes urine involuntarily in bed during sleep ≥ 1–2 times every week over at least 3 months). It is called secondary NE if the child had been dry by night continuously for more than 6 months and starts having this symptom. It may occur due to numerous causes:

1. Delayed maturation of nerve pathways for bladder control
2. Small capacity or overactive bladder
3. Deep sleep (prevents the child recognizing the sensation of bladder fullness)
4. Emotional or social stress (family discord, birth of a younger sibling).
5. Absence of the normal rise of antidiuretic hormone (ADH) level at night (ADH makes kidneys reabsorb more water and form less urine during night).

In some cases, the child appears well and enuresis could be the only symptom (monosymptomatic). The child may have many associated symptoms even during daytime (wetting). Dribbling, frequency, urgency, urine holding, infrequent voiding, straining to pass, pain on urination, constipation, fecal soiling or other problems (neuro-developmental) along with bed wetting (polysymptomatic). It is necessary to gather details about fluid intake patterns during day/night, amount and timing of bed-wetting and toileting behavior. If a child has secondary NE of recent onset, evaluation to rule out diseases like UTI and diabetes are necessary. Polysymptomatic NE with daytime symptoms need complete urinalysis, culture, blood tests and neurological evaluation. Children with bedwetting and emotional/behavioral problems need psychological evaluation and support.

Most children will learn to control their bladder habits by 7 years by bladder training exercises without drug treatment. Moisture detecting alarms in the undergarment is useful to alert the child at night. Waking of children by parents, either at regular times or randomly, is also a useful as a temporary practical measure. Alarm clock may be used to wake the older child at night. Use of caffeine-based drinks should be avoided. Drinking liquids after 6 pm may be restricted. Liberal fluid intake during daytime and inculcating the habit of timely voiding are helpful. The child is encouraged to pass urine at regular intervals during the day and just before sleep (typically 4–7 times/day). The drugs used are desmopressin, anticholinergic drugs, tricyclic antidepressants.

RENAL TUBULAR DISORDERS IN CHILDREN

In the kidney, the tubules reabsorb 99% of the glomerular filtrate. Reabsorption of Na^+, Cl^-, K^+, HCO_3^- (bicarbonate), glucose, calcium, magnesium, phosphates, amino acids and water as well as secretion of K^+ and H^+ ions (acid excretion) occur in various specialized parts of the tubule. Table 4.2 summarises important tubular disorders in children.

Tables 4.3 and 4.4 show the clinical features and investigations in various tubular disorders. For details, please see chapter on disorders of the renal tubule.

For the exact diagnosis of renal tubular disorders in children, timed or 24-hour urine collections are necessary. Special tests are done to measure the quantity urinary excretion of various substances (electrolytes, calcium, phosphate, citrate, oxalate, amino acids and uric acid).

Table 4.2: Summary of important tubular disorders in children

Part of tubule	Substance transported	Name of disease	Treatment
Proximal convoluted tubule (PCT)	HCO_3^-	Proximal RTA	Bicarbonate supplements
	Phosphate	Hypophosphatemic rickets	Phosphate and vitamin D
	Glucose	Renal glycosuria	None required
	Amino acids	Aminoacidurias	Variable
	All of the above	Fanconi syndrome	Na and KCl, citrate, bicarbonate and PO_4
Loop of Henle	Na^+, K^+, Cl^-	Bartter's syndrome	NaCl and KCl, NSAIDs
Distal (DCT)	H^+ ions (acid)	Distal RTA	Potassium citrate, bicarbonate
	Na^+, Cl^-	Gitelman syndrome	KCl, magnesium supplements
	Na^+, K^+	Liddle syndrome	Amiloride, low salt
Collecting duct	Na^+, K^+	Pseudohypoaldosteronism	K^+ restriction, salt supplements
	Water	Nephrogenic DI	Lot of water, NSAIDs, low salt

Note: Renal tubular acidosis (RTA); Diabetes insipidus (DI); Non-steroidal anti-inflammatory drugs (NSAIDs).

Table 4.3: Common clinical features of renal tubular disorders

Growth retardation, poor weight gain	Almost any tubular disorder
Polyuria, polydipsia, enuresis	Diabetes insipidus, Bartter's syndrome, RTAs, Fanconi syndrome
Preference for salty foods	Bartter's and Gitelman syndromes
Bony deformities, rickets	Hypophosphatemic rickets, RTAs
Hypertension	Liddle and other rarer disorders
Calcinosis of kidneys/stones in urine	Distal RTA, Bartter's syndrome, hypercalciurias

Table 4.4: Investigations for renal tubular diseases

Blood pH	Low	All types of RTAs	High	Bartter, Gitelman, Liddle
Serum HCO_3^-	Low	All RTAs, Fanconi	High	Bartter, Gitelman, Liddle
Serum Na^+	Low	Hypoaldosteronism	High	Diabetes insipidus
Serum K^+	Low	Bartter, Gitelman, Liddle, RTA	High	Hypoaldosteronism, Type 4 RTA
Serum Cl^-	Low	Bartter, Gitelman	High	All RTAs, DI
Others	Low	Serum magnesium in Gitelman	Low	Serum PO_4 in hypophosphatemic rickets

HIGH BLOOD PRESSURE—HYPERTENSION (HTN) IN CHILDREN

It is necessary to understand percentile. Percentile and percentage are different. For example, if a student scores 85/100 marks in an examination, his percentage mark is 85%. If it is the highest mark, his percentile score is 100%. It means, all the other students have scored less marks than this student. If a student's mark in the examination is in the 95th percentile, it means that 95% of those who took the examination got less marks than the student. In other words, he is in the top 5%.

In children, hypertension is defined as percentile values rather than numbers. The percentile curves were prepared (1987) based on age, height, weight and distributions of systolic and diastolic BP for infants and children. Diagnosis of hypertension can be made in children as per the following percentile values. (4th Task Force of The National Heart Lung and Blood Institute, USA.) All normal children will have BP below 90th percentile. If the BP is between 90th and 95th percentile, the condition is called pre-hypertension. If it is >95th percentile, it is Stage 1 hypertension and if the blood pressure is 5 mmHg >99th percentile, it is Stage 2. Any blood pressure >120/80 in an adolescent is hypertension. The approximate values for 95th percentile in various ages are (for exact values, please refer to the charts)

1 year = 105/58,

6 years = 115/75,

12 years = 125/80 and

18 years = 130/85.

Etiology: Common causes of hypertension in children of various ages are given in Table 4.5.

Table 4.5: Common causes of hypertension in children of various age groups

Infants	1–6 years	7–12 years	Adolescent
Thrombosis of renal artery or vein Congenital renal	Renal artery stenosis Renal parenchymal disease	Renal parenchymal disease (e.g. nephritis) Renovascular abnormalities	Essential hypertension Renal parenchymal disease
Coarctation of aorta Bronchopulmonary dysplasia	Wilms' tumor Neuroblastoma coarctation of aorta	Endocrine causes Essential hypertension	Endocrine causes

Treatment

In secondary HTN, the primary cause should be treated. Other measures for BP control similar to those used in essential (primary) HTN may be required for all. Non-pharmacologic measures alone may be sufficient for moderate elevations of BP. Weight control, exercise—aerobic and isotonic, low salt-low fat, potassium-rich diet, stress-reducing activities (meditation, yoga, biofeedback) are major non-pharmacologic measures. Pharmacologic measures include use of antihypertensive medications similar to those used in adults.

KIDNEY FAILURE IN CHILDREN

The term 'Kidney failure' implies significant reduction in glomerular filtration rate (GFR). GFR in children is usually calculated by the Schwartz formula as given in the box below.

Schwartz Formula

$$eGFR \, (ml/min/1.73 \, m^2) = \frac{k \times (Height \, in \, cm)}{Serum \, creatinine \, in \, mg/dl}$$

[k = A constant; its value varies with age]

- k = 0.33 in premature infants up to 1 year of age
- k = 0.45 in term infants up to 1 year of age
- k = 0.55 in children 2 to 13 years of age and in adolescent females up to 18 years
- k = 0.70 in adolescent males (because of the presumed increase of muscle mass in males)

ACUTE KIDNEY INJURY (AKI) AND ACUTE RENAL FAILURE (ARF)

AKI is defined as rapid deterioration (within hours to days) of renal function to such an extent that the kidneys cannot regulate fluid and electrolyte homeostasis. It is often reversible. The classification of AKI in adults and pediatric patients is slightly different. A classification system called RIFLE criteria (*R*: Risk for renal dysfunction, *I*: Injury to the kidney, *F*: Failure of kidney function, *L*: Loss of kidney function, and *E*: End-stage renal disease), originally proposed for standardized AKI classification in adults is adapted for pediatric patients as pediatric RIFLE (pRIFLE) (Table 4.6).

Table 4.6: RIFLE' classification of AKI

pRIFLE scale	Estimated creatinine clearance (eCCl)	Urine output
Risk	eCCl decrease by 25%	<0.5 ml/kg/hr for 8 hrs
Injury	eCCl decrease by 50%	<0.5 ml/kg/hr for 16 hrs
Failure	eCCl decrease by 75% or is <35 ml/min/1.73 m²	<0.5 ml/kg/hr for 24 hrs or Anuric for ≥12 hrs
Loss	Persistent failure >4 weeks	
End stage	Persistent failure >3 months	

Note: From kidney international 2007; 71:1028–35

(The eCCl in this classification is same as the eGFR calculated by the Schwartz formula).

Etiology: AKI can be divided into pre-renal causes, intrinsic renal causes and obstructive causes. Some causes such as cortical necrosis and renal vein thrombosis are more common in neonates, hemolytic uremic syndrome (HUS) in young children, and rapidly progressive GN (RPGN) generally in older children and adolescents. The common causes in children are shown in Table 4.7.

Table 4.7: Common causes of AKI in children

Type	Etiology	Common causes in children
Prerenal	Low true intravascular volume	Diarrhea, shock—dengue, sepsis, cardiac surgery
	Low effective intravascular volume	Cardiac failure
Intrinsic renal	Acute tubular necrosis (vasomotor nephropathy)	Hypoxia/ischemia, drugs, tumor lysis syndrome, toxins—exogenous (snake venom)/endogenous
	Interstitial nephritis	Drug induced idiopathic
	Glomerulonephritis	RPGN
	Vascular lesions	Renal artery/vein thrombosis, cortical necrosis microvascular thrombosis—HUS
	Hypoplasia/dysplasia	Idiopathic, exposure to nephrotoxic drugs *in utero*
Postrenal	Obstructive uropathy	Obstruction in a solitary kidney/both ureters or urethra by calculi, clots, etc.

The steps in the management are similar to general principles as in adults except that fluid management is more difficult in children and they may require dialysis support earlier as compared to adults. Acute peritoneal dialysis is used more commonly in children with AKI who need dialysis.

CHRONIC KIDNEY DISEASE (CKD) AND CHRONIC RENAL FAILURE (CRF)

CKD and CRF are not the same. CKD means there is some abnormality in the kidney persistently for more than 3 months. The GFR may or may not be abnormal in early stages. (See classification in the chapter on CKD.) The abnormality can be any one of the following.

1. Kidney damage: Structural or functional abnormalities of the kidney (with or without decreased GFR):
   a. Abnormalities in blood or urine test results
   b. Abnormalities in imaging tests
   c. Abnormalities on kidney biopsy
   d. GFR <60 ml/min/1.73 m^2 for 3 months.

CKD can be present at any age, even in neonatal period or infancy. If an infant is born with congenital abnormality, it is called CKD even if the GFR is normal for the age. Similarly, if there is a urinary abnormality of abnormal blood test of kidney function for more than 3 months, the condition can be called CKD. Some kidney diseases that are congenital or start during childhood can progress to end-stage renal disease (ESRD) in late childhood or adulthood. CKD in children could be due to congenital or acquired causes (Table 4.8).

Table 4.8: Common causes of CKD in children

Congenital disorders	Acquired disorders
1. Malformations/developmental disorders: Renal hypoplasia, dysplasia, obstructive uropathy Neurogenic bladder	**1. Glomerulonephritis:** Focal segmental glomerulosclerosis Crescentic GN Membranoproliferative GN
2. Hereditary/congenital disorders: Nephronophthisis polycystic kidney disease, Alport's syndrome Congenital nephrotic syndrome	**2. Thrombotic microangiopathy,** e.g. hemolytic uremic syndrome
	3. Chronic pyelonephritis with/ without VU reflux
	4. Miscellaneous: Interstitial nephritis

CRF is state of irreversible kidney damage with low GFR which has been present for >3 months. This condition may remain as such or progress to end-stage renal disease (ESRD).

MANAGEMENT OF CKD IN CHILDREN

1. Confirm diagnosis and classify as glomerular or tubulo-interstitial.
   a. Glomerular diseases are associated with heavy proteinuria, presence of red blood cells and casts in urine, high BP, edema and reduced urine output.
   b. Tubulointerstitial disorders are associated with minimal proteinuria, unremarkable urine sediments except for pus cells if associated with UTI, polyuria, absence of edema and often bony deformities. BP may be variable depending on the underlying cause.
2. Try to identify primary cause (see Table 4.8) if possible. It may not be possible if patient presents in end-stage with small shrunken kidneys.
3. Check for co-morbidities in other systems.
4. Look for reversible/correctable factors
   a. Hypertension
   b. Infections
   c. Urinary tract obstruction
   d. Stones
   e. Use of nephrotoxic drugs
   f. Severe proteinuria and
   g. Poor glycemic control in diabetics
5. Adequate nutrition and promoting growth
6. Correct hydration—fluid overload/dehydration
7. Correct mineral and bone disorder (CKD-MBD—renal osteodystrophy), electrolyte abnormalities and acidosis
8. Treat/control uremic complications—gastropathy, encephalopathy, pericarditis, neuropathy, itching.
9. Prevent progression (evaluate and manage risk factors for progression)
10. Plan for timely renal replacement therapy.

Conservative Management

1. Specific therapy of primary disease (if a treatable cause is detected)
2. Manage co-morbidities

3. Prevent and treat complications
   a. Maintain adequate nutrition and growth
   b. Fluid, electrolyte and acid–base balance—intake regulated low/high based on type of CKD, judicious use of diuretics
   c. Anemia management—iron, erythropoietin injections
   d. BP control
   e. Management of CKD-MBD—vitamin D and calcium supplements, phosphate control
   f. Immunisations—check hepatitis B antibody titres and vaccinate with double dose if low
   g. Measures to slow progression to ESRD
4. Regular follow-up
5. Early preparation for kidney failure and renal replacement therapy (dialysis/renal transplant). Peritoneal dialysis is preferable to hemodialysis in infants, toddlers and most children. Transplantation in small children <15–20 kg weight is technically challenging.

5

Importance of Urine Examination

Dhanya Binu, R Kasi Visweswaran

Urine examination is the first and most simple test to diagnose diseases of the kidneys or urinary system. Early morning sample is usually taken. The method of urine collection must be proper. About 50–100 ml of urine is collected into a clean dry container. Midstream clean catch urine is preferred. In the case of males, the prepuce should be retracted and cleaned so that the urine flows directly from the tip of the urethra to the sample container. In the case of females, the external genitalia is cleaned and labia is held separated so that the urine flows directly from the tip of the urethra to the sample container.

In women, urine examination particularly for blood/microscopy should be avoided during menstrual cycles. In women during periods or in children, the urine sample may be obtained by single use catheter (only if absolutely necessary). Collecting urine samples from an indwelling catheter or urinary bag should be preferably avoided.

For collecting timed sample of 6, 8, 12 or 24 hrs, the patient is asked to empty the bladder at the time of starting collection which should be discarded. Thereafter all the urine passed should be collected into the container till the specified time at 6, 8, 12 or 24 hrs. For example, if the patient is to collect a 24-hour urine sample from 6 am to 6 am the next day, the patient should be instructed to empty the bladder at 6 am on the first day and discard the sample. Thereafter all the urine passed including the final collection at 6 am the next day should be collected cleanly and transferred to container or directly into the container.

In children, sample for urine culture may be taken through supra-pubic needle puncture into a full bladder. In this case, the syringe with the needle capped may be taken directly to the laboratory. In children, urine collecting devices attached to external genitalia may be used for collecting samples. In adult males with incontinence, condom catheters may be used to collect urine for routine tests. These samples may not be suitable for cultures. Collecting urine samples for culture by disconnecting indwelling catheter is not reliable since contaminants grow in it. In indwelling catheters, a 'bio-film' is formed after a few days and organisms may grow in them. If urine samples for culture are necessary from a patient on indwelling catheter, it is advisable to remove the indwelling catheter, use a new catheter and take a sample immediately. This will avoid the contamination due to the bio-film. If there is any undue delay in sending for culture, the sample should be refrigerated. If there is likely to be a delay in microscopic examination, 1 drop of formalin in 30 ml urine may be added. Obtaining a urine sample from the urinary bag should be discouraged.

When 24-hour urine specimens have to be collected, it is mandatory that a preservative is added to the container in order to prevent decomposition and growth of microorganisms. Preservatives are necessary if the samples are to be transported to a distant laboratory. For culture and sensitivity midstream urine sample is collected into a sterile container directly and must be closed immediately. Steps to correctly handle the container should be explained to the patient.

In order to identify the source of turbidity/hematuria, the whole of urine passed is collected into 3 large sample bottles as follows. The initial portion of the urinary stream is collected in container 1, middle portion in 2 and last portion in 3. If the initial portion (sample 1) is blood stained, the source of bleeding is from the urethra. If the terminal portion of the urine flow alone (sample 3) is cloudy/blood stained, it suggests lesions in the urinary bladder or trigone. If all the 3 samples are uniformly turbid/blood stained, it suggests that the urine remaining in the bladder is already cloudy/blood stained.

The container is labeled correctly and sent to the laboratory with the correct, completed request form.

MACROSCOPIC EXAMINATION OF URINE

Volume

The normal urine output ranges from 1200 to 2000 ml/day. Polyuria is the term used when the 24-hour urine output exceeds 3000 ml.

Polyuria is seen after excessive fluid intake, in cold weather conditions and diseases like diabetes insipidus and diabetes mellitus. Oliguria is the term used when the 24-hour urine output decreases below 500 ml. Oliguria may be seen in hot climates, decreased fluid intake and in various stages of kidney diseases. Anuria refers to the urinary output less than 100 ml in 24 hours to total absence of urine output. If a patient does not pass even a few drops of urine, obstruction to the urinary tract should be suspected.

Color of Urine

Normal freshly passed urine is pale yellow/straw colored. The color of normal urine is due to a pigment called urochrome and small amounts of urobilin which is present in it. In cold climate or following adequate water intake, the urine may be almost like water and if the person has not taken adequate water and the climate is hot, the urine may have dark 'amber' color. The color of freshly passed urine may be different in some diseases or following intake of drugs or dyes. Table 5.1 summarizes the causes of changes in color of urine. In some conditions, the color of freshly passed urine may be normal but the color may change after a few hours. This is common in a genetic condition called alkaptonuria; where the cloth which has come into contact with urine gets a permanent dark brownish stain. Presence of bilirubin imparts a golden brown/orange yellow, conjugated bilirubin, greenish yellow and unconjugated bilirubin lemon yellow color to urine (Table 5.1).

Table 5.1: Some common causes of abnormal color of urine

Color	Disease	Drugs
Pink/red/orange	Hematuria	Phenazopyridine (pyridium, beetroot, rifampicin, phenytoin)
Brown/black	Phenylketonuria, melanin pigment after sometime	Nitrofurantoin, metronidazole, iron sortibol
Blue/green, greenish yellow	Obstructive jaundice	Triamterene
Red/reddish brown/cola colored	Acute nephritis, hematuria, hemoglobinuria, myoglobinuria	
White/milk/cloudy	Chyluria, pyuria	

Appearance

Normal urine is clear. If amorphous phosphates are present and they precipitate and urine may turn turbid on storage. Mucus, prostatic secretion or amorphous urates may cause urine to become cloudy. Urinary tract infection is the commonest disease causing cloudy urine. Diseases causing chyluria *(lymph in urine)* may also lead to cloudy urine. Sterile pyuria is the disease condition when a patient has persistent pyuria, but the bacterial cultures are sterile and this is common in genitourinary tuberculosis.

Odor

Freshly passed urine is odorless. It develops the characteristic ammoniac odor on exposure to air when the urea is split into ammonia by the bacteria. If freshly passed urine (without contamination from external genitalia) is 'foul smelling', it suggests bacterial infection of the urinary tract.

Reaction

The reaction of urine is usually acidic. The pH measures the acidity or alkalinity of urine. Normally it varies between pH 4.5 and 8.0. The pH of urine is important in diagnosis of disorders of renal tubule like renal tubular acidosis. Urine pH can be modified by administration of acidic or alkaline substances or use of some drugs like sulfonamides, allopurinol. For acidification of urine vitamin C can be used, for alkalinisation; citrate or bicarbonates can be used. In conditions like crystalluria due to oxalate or uric acid crystals alkalinisation of urine will help. In some types of infection acidification of urine may be beneficial. Some drugs act better in acid urine.

Specific Gravity

The specific gravity of normal urine varies from 1.005 to 1.025. It is measured by using a urinometer. When the urine is dilute, the specific gravity is lesser than 1.010. The specific gravity of the glomerular filtrate is 1.010. In chronic renal failure the specific gravity of urine may be around 1.010 irrespective of the body's condition. This type of 'fixed' specific gravity is called 'isosthenuria'. During water deprivation test, the specific gravity should increase to >1.016. In spite of water deprivation, if the urinary specific gravity remains <1.005, it suggests diabetes insipidus (DI).

If the DI is central in type, administration of the pituitary hormone vasopressin helps to improve the specific gravity to >1.016. In nephrogenic DI, the vasopressin is present in the body but is not able to act on the renal tubules. Therefore, there will be no improvement in urinary specific gravity in spite of administration of vasopressin.

The osmolality of urine varies from 50 to 1200 mOsm/kg. Dilute urine is associated with lower osmolality and concentrated urine has osmolality >450 mOsm/kg. The osmolality in "isosthenuria" is around 300 mOsm/kg. Urine osmolality can be calculated from urinary sodium potassium, urea and ammonia or is measured using an instrument called 'osmometer'. The osmometer measures the osmolality from the freezing point of the test solution.

CHEMICAL EXAMINATION OF URINE

Proteins in Urine

Some protein is lost in the urine under normal conditions. The normal daily urinary protein excretion is between 150 and 300 mg. This consists of Tamm-Horsfall protein secreted by the renal tubule, immunoglobulin and beta-2 microglobulin.

In diseases of glomeruli, the proteins including albumin from blood are filtered and cannot be reabsorbed completely. Therefore, the urine examination shows 3+ to 4+ protein when heated in a test tube. Dipstix for albumin are commonly used and the result analysed based on the change in color as 1 to 4+. Quantity of protein excreted in urine can be assessed by doing 24-hour urine protein estimation, or by assessing the ratio of urinary protein and creatinine (urine protein creatinine ratio). Bence Jones proteinuria is excretion of a part of immunoglobulin in urine. This occurs in multiple myeloma. Testing for microalbuminuria is done to detect very small quantities of albumin in urine. This may occur in very early stages of diabetic nephropathy. Test for microalbuminuria should be done only when diabetes and hypertension are well controlled. Patient should not suffer from fever, urinary tract infection or undertake heavy physical activity. The test can be done in a properly collected 24-hour sample or by doing urine albumin creatinine ratio.

The normal urinary microalbumin is < 30 mg/day. When it is between 30 and 300 mg/day, it is called microalbuminuria. When it is > 300 mg, it can be easily diagnosed even without microalbuminuria test since the regular urine tests like albustix or heat coagulation test will be positive.

Sugar in Urine

Normally, the glucose in the blood that is filtered by the glomerulus is fully reabsorbed by the tubule. Therefore, no glucose is excreted through urine. Glucose starts to appear in urine (glycosuria) only when the plasma glucose level exceeds the capacity of the tubule to reabsorb. When the blood sugar level is >180–200 mg/dl, glycosuria occurs. Uncontrolled diabetes mellitus is the most common cause of glycosuria. Other diseases like thyrotoxicosis, Cushing's syndrome, increased intracranial pressure, intravenous infusion of glucose may also cause high blood sugar level leading to glycosuria. Many drugs can cause increase in blood sugar level and glycosuria (e.g. steroids). In alimentary glycosuria, the blood level goes up immediately after food and there may be transient glycosuria.

Sometimes, the capacity of the renal tubule to reabsorb glucose may be defective. In these cases, glucose will appear in urine even though the blood sugar level is normal. This condition is called renal glycosuria. Some congenital diseases or drugs can affect the function of tubules resulting in renal glycosuria. If the ability of the tubule to reabsorb other substances is also affected, there will be defective reabsorption of phosphate, bicarbonate, amino acids, etc. This condition is referred to as Fanconi's syndrome.

The conventional urine test for sugar may be positive when reducing substances other than glucose that may be seen in urine. Presence of lactose, pentose, fructose, galactose, homogentisic acid, ascorbic acid, dextrin, and proteins may produce a false positive result on routine urine examination. They can be differentiated by special tests. Benedict's test is the most commonly used test for glucosuria. Now dipstix for glucose are available. Glucose oxidase method using glucostix or clinistix is the most reliable and specific test for glucose. Currently, serial blood sugar levels are done to monitor blood sugar.

Ketone Bodies in Urine

Ketone bodies are products of incomplete fat metabolism. Three chemical compounds: Acetone, acetoacetic acid and betahydroxy butyric acid are the common keto acids. These substances are produced by liver from free fatty acids. Accumulation of these substances in blood is known as ketoacidosis. If ketone bodies are present in urine, it is called ketonuria. Ketonuria is seen in uncontrolled diabetes mellitus, prolonged starvation, eclampsia, prolonged vomiting, severe diarrhea and in glycogen storage disorders. The tests done for testing ketone bodies is Rothera's test. It can be done with Acetest or ketotest strip method also.

Bile in Urine

Urochromes and small amounts of urobilin are found in urine under normal circumstances. Breakdown products of hemoglobin such as bilirubin, urobilinogen and urobilin as well as bile salts will be excreted in urine in certain abnormal conditions.

Hemoglobin is broken down into bilirubin, metabolized (conjugation) in the liver and is excreted into the bile. If there is obstruction to the flow of bile or there is damage to the liver cells, the conjugated bilirubin enters into the systemic circulation and will be excreted in the urine. When the conjugated bilirubin reaches the intestine, it is acted upon by the intestinal bacteria and converted to urobilinogen. Most of this urobilinogen is converted into stercobilinogen and is excreted in the feces. A portion of urobilinogen is reabsorbed and excreted through urine. Hence, trace amounts of urobilinogen can be found in normal urine. In obstructive jaundice (obstruction of the bile duct), there will be no urobilinogen in urine.

Jaundice is a clinical sign that develops when there is yellowish pigmentation of the skin and mucous membrane due to deposition of bile pigments. When there is an increase in the breakdown of hemoglobin such as in hemolytic anemia or when there is hepatocellular damage, there is increase in urobilinogen in urine. Bilirubinuria is seen when excess of conjugated or water-soluble form of bilirubin is excreted in urine. This occurs in hepatocellular damage which causes intrahepatic bile duct obstruction and also in other causes of bile duct obstruction.

Therefore, testing for both urobilinogen and bilirubin in urine is important in evaluating a patient with jaundice.

Urobilinogen is detected in urine by Ehrlich's test or dipstix. Bilirubin can be detected by Fouchet's test or dipstix. Bile salts appear in urine only if obstruction to their excretion in bile occurs. Bile salts can be tested by Hay's test.

Blood or Hemoglobin in Urine

Hematuria is the term used where intact RBC (>10 RBC/HPF) is found in the urine sample. Urine may show presence of intact RBC if samples have been taken from a woman during menstrual cycles. This is due to contamination with menstrual blood. Hematuria can be due to diseases in the kidney, stones, tumors, infections, injury or following operations in the urinary tract. Renal causes include neoplasm, calculi, tuberculosis of kidney, pyelonephritis, acute glomerulonephritis and congenital cystic diseases. Postrenal causes include ureteric calculus, bilharziasis, tuberculosis, malignant hypertension, malaria, neoplasm of the urinary tract.

Hemoglobinuria is the term used when hemoglobin is present in urine. This is due to the destruction of RBCs in the vascular system (intravascular hemolysis). Free hemoglobin in the plasma binds to haptoglobin in the blood. When excessive free hemoglobin is present, it is excreted by the kidneys. Hemoglobin in urine forms crystals in the tubules if the urine is acidic. Therefore, whenever hemoglobinuria is suspected, the patient is given alkai to help the urine to become alkaline in reaction. Hemoglobinuria is seen in malaria, hemolytic streptococcal infection, drug intake, incompatible blood transfusion and paroxysmal nocturnal hemoglobinuria. In a deficiency of the RBC enzyme called glucose-6-phosphate dehydrogenase (G6PD deficiency), massive hemolysis may occur when the patient is given some drugs (e.g. paracetamol, chloroquine). G6PD deficiency is common in some families and communities.

It is important to distinguish between hematuria and hemoglobinuria. If the macroscopic examination of the urine sample is reddish, the sample has to be centrifuged, if the supernatant is reddish in colour it is due to hemoglobinuria and if the sediment is reddish it is due to hematuria. In hematuria, the sediment will show RBCs under the microscope. To detect hemoglobin in urine, benzidine test is used. Dipstick test or immunochemical method by nephelometry also may be used.

Microscopic Examination of Urine

Examination of urine sediments under the microscope is one of the most important tests that can be done to evaluate diseases of kidney and urinary tract. Urine sediments are obtained by centrifugation of 10 ml of fresh urine sample at 1500 rpm for 5 minutes. They are divided into two types—unorganized sediments and organized sediments.

Unorganized sediments include mainly crystals (Table 5.2 and Fig. 5.1).

Crystals are formed by the precipitation of urinary salts depending on various factors like pH of urine, concentration of urine and drug administration.

Line diagram of some crystals is shown in Fig. 5.1.

Organized substances in urine include red blood cells, leucocytes, yeasts, trichomonas vaginalis, spermatozoa, epithelial cells, casts, eggs or larvae of parasites.

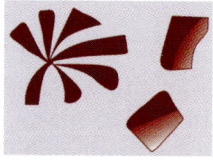

Uric acid crystal

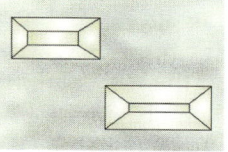

Triple phosphate ('coffin lid' appearance)

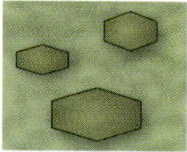

Cystine crystals

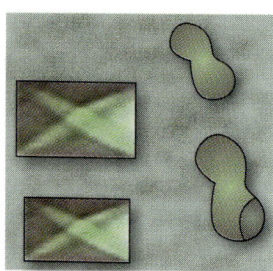

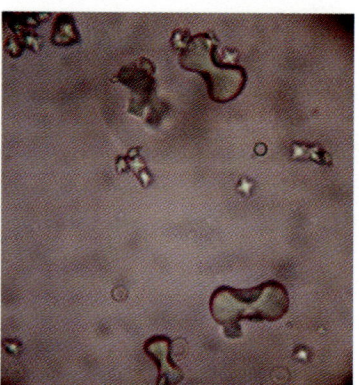

Calcium oxalate (envelop shaped or dumbell shaped crystals)

Fig. 5.1: Shapes of some common crystals

Table 5.2: Crystals found in urine	
Crystals in acidic urine	Crystals in alkaline urine
Uric acid and urates	Ammonium magnesium phosphates
Calcium oxalates	Dicalcium phosphates
Cystine	Calcium carbonate
Leucine and tyrosine	Ammonium biurate
Sulpha crystals	

These are long transparent cylindrical structures whose presence in urine indicates renal diseases. The main component of the cast is 'Tamm-Horsfall' protein which is secreted by the tubules. It forms a cylindrical mould of the tubular lumen and is passed. If there are cells or fat in the tubular lumen, they are included within the cast. Different types of cast may have different significance (Fig. 5.2 and Table 5.3).

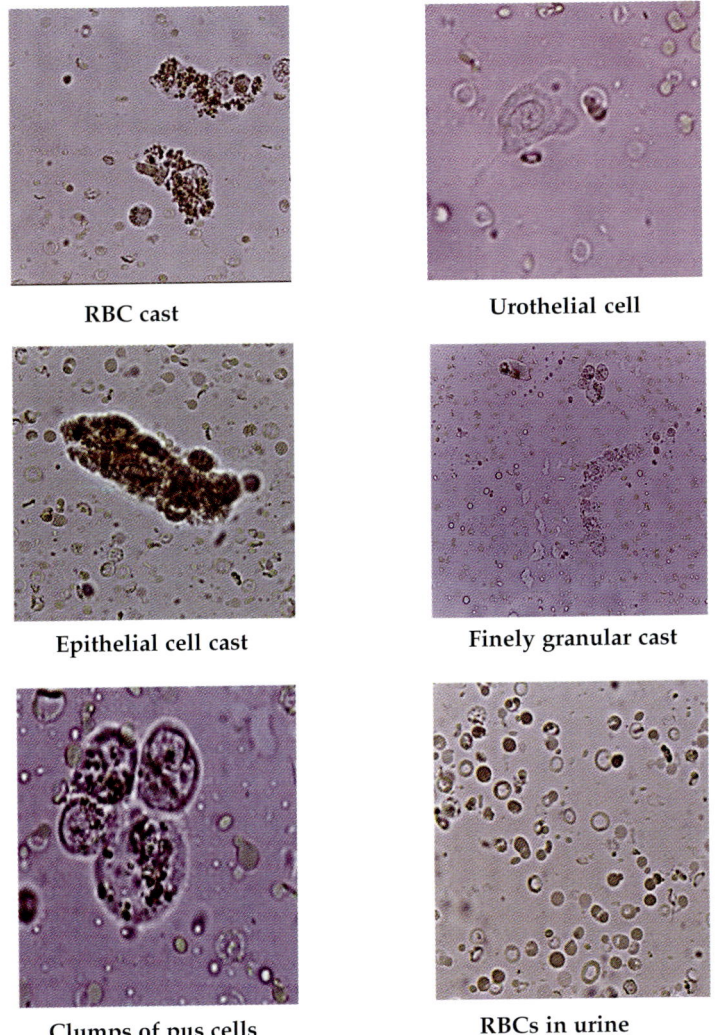

RBC cast

Urothelial cell

Epithelial cell cast

Finely granular cast

Clumps of pus cells

RBCs in urine

Fig. 5.2: Urine microscopy of cells and casts

Table 5.3: Different types of casts and their significance

Casts	Appearance	Disease conditions
Hyaline casts	Colorless, transparent	Glomerulonephritis
Epithelial casts	Filled with pale yellow cells	Tubular damage
Granular casts	Short, studded with degenerated cells	Glomerulonephritis
Fatty casts	Yellowish and refractile, minimal change	Diabetic nephropathy glomerulonephritis
Waxy casts	Light yellow, refractile	Advanced glomerulonephritis
RBC casts	Brownish	Acute glomerulonephritis
Leucocyte casts	Casts studded with leucocytes	Pyelonephritis

BIBLIOGRAPHY

1. John Bernard Henry, *Clinical Diagnosis and Management by Laboratory Methods;* 20th edition.
2. Robert H Carman, *Handbook of Medical Laboratory Technology.*

6

Blood Investigations in Kidney Disease

Satheesh Balakrishnan, R Kasi Visweswaran

When renal disease is suspected, detailed history is recorded followed by physical examination and simple urine tests are performed first. Later, other investigations are planned according to the illness or syndrome suspected. The basic blood tests and special blood investigations to diagnose kidney diseases are discussed in this chapter.

BASIC TESTS

Blood examination is done to assess hemoglobin, total WBC count, differential count, erythrocyte sedimentation rate (ESR), packed cell volume (PCV) and examination of peripheral blood smear. Hemoglobin is generally low in chronic renal failure. This could be due to deficiency of iron, vitamin B_{12}, folic acid or erythropoietin (EPO). EPO is a hormone produced in the kidney which stimulates the bone marrow to produce RBCs. Anemia due to renal failure is often due to deficiency of EPO. Although the hemoglobin level is low, the size and amount of hemoglobin in each red cell will be normal when examined by blood smear (normocytic normochromic blood picture). The total and differential leucocyte count may be abnormal in most infections. Very high erythrocyte sedimentation rate is observed in conditions like collagen disorders, multiple myeloma or malignancies. Examination of the peripheral blood smear may reveal normocytic normochromic anemia, microangiopathic hemolytic anemia or thrombocytopenia. A combination of anemia, leucopenia and thrombocytopenia may be seen in collagen vascular diseases.

Urea is an end product of protein metabolism and is excreted in the urine. The blood contains 20–40 mg% of urea. If the kidney function is deranged, the urea level increases. The blood urea level is expressed as mg% or mmol/L depending on the method used in the laboratory for testing. There is a fixed relationship between the mg% and mmol/L for each substance. In the case of urea, 60 mg% = 10 mmol/L. Some laboratories measure only the nitrogen in the urea molecule and express the result as blood urea nitrogen (BUN). There is a fixed relationship between BUN and blood urea but BUN and urea are not the same. Blood urea 60 mg% = BUN 28. For all clinical puroposes, BUN can be taken as 50% of urea. The urea level increases when the kidney function is poor. Accumulation of waste products including urea results in the symptoms of uremia. The blood level of urea may increase due to high protein intake in the diet, dehydration or oliguria. The level of urea can come down due to poor food intake, overhydration or polyuria. Low urea level indicates poor nutrition and negative nitrogen balance.

Creatinine is an end product of muscle breakdown. The normal level of serum creatinine varies between males and females. Those who are muscular have a slightly higher creatinine compared to lean or less muscular individuals. The normal values vary from 0.8 to 1.2 mg%. Serum creatinine is measured in micromoles/L in the SI system. 1.0 mg% creatinine = 88.5 micromoles/L. The level of creatinine does not change significantly with high or low protein diet. If the kidney functions are stable, the serum creatinine levels remain steady. It gives an idea about glomerular filtration rate (GFR). When the serum creatinine level doubles, the GFR reduces by 50%. In acute kidney injury, the serum creatinine rises by 0.5 to 1.0 mg% per day. If the kidney injury is severe and is associated with muscle injury or traffic accident, the creatinine may rise by even 2 mg% per day. This condition is called hypercatabolic renal failure and such patients may require more intensive dialysis.

Glomerular filtration rate (GFR) is an index of renal function. It can be measured by checking 24-hour sample of urine for creatinine, serum creatinine and calculating creatinine clearance. Rough estimate of glomerular filtration can be made at the bedside with some calculations.

a. Reciprocal of creatinine value: For approximate % of kidney function
1/serum creatinine × 100 gives approximate % of renal function.
Example: Serum creatinine 3 mg% → 1 × 100/3 = 33.33% kidney function.
Serum creatinine 5 mg% → 1 × 100/5 = 20% kidney function.

b. Cockcroft Gault formula:

This formula takes into consideration, age, body weight and serum creatinine level. It is not reliable in children.

Adult males → eGFR (ml/min)

$$= \frac{[140 - (\text{age in years})] \times \text{body weight (kg)}}{72 \times \text{serum creatinine (mg\%)}}$$

Adult females → eGFR (ml/min)

$$= \frac{[140 - (\text{age in years})] \times \text{body weight (kg)}}{72 \times \text{serum creatinine (mg\%)}} \times 0.85$$

c. Modification of diet in renal disease (MDRD) equation and chronic kidney disease epidemiology (CKD EPI) equations are more complex and take into consideration age, gender, race into consideration. CKD EPI equation is more reliable compared to MDRD if the GFR is more than 60 ml/min. Now, online and offline programs or calculators are available for these calculations.

Uric acid in the serum is an end product of purine metabolism and is excreted by the kidneys. The normal levels are between 4–6 mg% in males and 3.5–5.0 mg% in females. The uric acid level may increase as a result of renal failure, errors in uric acid metabolism or as a result of overproduction in the body. During chemotherapy/radiation treatment of malignancies, cancer cells are killed in large numbers. The nuclear remnants contain purines which are metabolized to uric acid and sudden increase in uric acid level occurs. This may lead to acute gout or acute kidney injury.

Serum electrolytes usually tested are sodium, potassium and bicarbonate. Serum chloride estimation is also necessary for calculating anion gap and assessing metabolic alkalosis. The normal value for serum sodium is 135–145 mmol/L. Values below 135 suggest hyponatremia and more than 145 hypernatremia. Serum potassium is a very important investigation in renal disease. The normal blood level is between 3.5 and 5.0 mmol/L. Serum bicarbonate levels vary between 24 and 26 mmol/L and chloride levels 90–105 mmol/L. (Please refer to the respective chapters in the electrolyte and acid–base section.)

SERUM CALCIUM, PHOSPHORUS AND ALKALINE PHOSPHATASE

The normal level of serum calcium is between 9 and 11 mg%. If it is more than 11.5, the condition is called hypercalcemia and less than 8 mg% hypocalcemia. The serum calcium decreases in renal failure and is high in conditions like multiple myeloma and hyperparathyroidism. The normal level of serum phosphorus is between 2.5 and 4.5 mg%. Dietary phosphorus is absorbed and is excreted by the kidneys. Phosphorus is necessary for cellular functions and formation of bone. When the kidney function fails, phosphorus accumulates in the blood leading to hyperphosphatemia. Diet low in phosphates is advised for such patients. Phosphate binding drugs like calcium acetate, calcium carbonate, sevelemer or Lanthanum carbonate are administered with food so that these drugs bind with the phosphorus in the gut and prevent its absorption. Hypophosphatemia can occur as a result of the inability of the renal tubule to reabsorb the filtered phosphate leading to loss of phosphates in the urine and hypophosphatemia. (see chapter on electrolytes in Section 2). Alkaline phosphatase is an enzyme and the blood level varies from 40 to 140 international units/L. It is often elevated in bone diseases and liver diseases. Alkaline phosphatase may be higher than normal in biliary obstruction, bone diseases, liver diseases, hyperparathyroidism and rickets. It is lower in hypophosphatasia and malnutrition. In renal failure, high alkaline phosphatase denotes bone involvement.

SERUM PROTEINS

The normal level of total proteins in the serum is 6.0 to 8.0 gm%. Although the plasma contains albumin, globulins and fibrinogen, the serum contains only albumin and globulins because fibrinogen is used up during clotting of blood. Normally, blood contains 4.0 to 6.0 gm% of albumin. Serum albumin is a good indicator of nutritional status. In conditions like nephrotic syndrome, malnutrition or liver disease, the serum albumin level will be very low. The globulins consist of alpha, beta 1, beta 2 and gamma globulins. It is possible to identify the different types of globulins by electrophoresis of serum. Gammaglobulins are the immunoglobulins (Igs). For identifying different types of gamma-globulins, immune-electrophoresis is used. Proteins of the Ig family are involved in antibody response. IgG, IgA, IgM, IgD and IgE are the subtypes of the Igs. Usually, the total serum proteins, albumin and globulins are measured and the albumin–globulin ratio (AG ratio) is calculated. The AG ratio varies from 1.5 : 1 to 2.0 : 1. When the ratio is reverse of normal, it is called AG reversal. AG reversal occurs when the albumin decreases or the globulin increases or both.

LIPID PROFILE

Cholesterol, triglycerides and chylomicrons are the usual types of lipids in the serum. Lipid profile should be checked in the fasting state since the level of lipids increase after food because of absorption from the gut. Abnormalities in the lipid profile are seen in many diseases and the pattern is different. In some conditions, the cholesterol alone may be elevated. Then it is called hypercholesterolemia. When triglycerides are increased, the condition is called hypertriglyceridemia. Patients with nephrotic syndrome, chronic renal failure, those on dialysis or those after renal transplantation have different patterns of hyperlipidemia.

Other special blood tests done for diagnosis of various kidney diseases are:

1. **Serum (intact) PTH level:** Done in patients with renal failure or maintenance dialysis to see the activity of parathyroid gland.

2. **Serum iron, total iron binding capacity and ferritin:** These tests are done to study if the body iron stores and iron metabolism within the body are normal. They are done before starting intravenous iron and erythropoietin therapy.

3. **Vitamin D level:** Because of nutritional factors and poor exposure to direct sunlight, most persons are vitamin D deficient. Simple vitamin D deficiency will respond to cholecalciferol. In renal failure, the patients need replacement of vitamin D with active 1, 25-dihydroxyvitamin D.

4. **Antistreptolysin O (ASO):** To diagnose recent infection with streptococci.

5. **Anti-DNAse B:** Another test to look for antibodies Group A Streptococcus.

6. **Antihyaluronidase:** Antibodies to streptococcal antigen or for rheumatic fever.

7. **Hepatitis B:** Hepatitis B surface antigen (HbsAg) is a screening test to diagnose hepatitis B infection.

8. **Anti-HCV antibody:** Screening test for hepatitis C infection

9. **HIV screening test:** Screening for infection with HIV.

10. **CMV antibody test:** Testing for prior exposure or active infection with cytomegalovirus. IgM and IgG antibodies to CMV are tested by enzyme-linked immunosorbent assay (ELISA). Positive test for CMV IgG indicates that a person was infected with CMV at some time during his life. Single

IgG test cannot determine when a person was infected. If antibody tests done during acute- and convalescent-phase show a four-fold rise in IgG antibody and CMV IgM antibody is also present or CMV virus is cultured from a urine or throat specimen, an active CMV infection is diagnosed.

11. Epstein-Barr virus antibody test—done to confirm infection with EB virus.

12. Antineutrophil cytoplasmic antibodies (ANCA)—pANCA and cANCA are tests to diagnose various types of vasculitis.

13. Antiglomerular basement membrane antibody (antiGBM Ab), to diagnose diseases like Goodpasture syndrome in which the body produces antibodies against the glomerular basement membrane.

14. Serum complement levels—CH 50 (total complement) = 40–90 units. C3 = 60–200 mg%.

15. These values may be variable and the laboratory ranges should be considered.

16. Antinuclear antibody (ANA)/anti-double-stranded DNA antibody (anti-dsDNA Ab)/antiphospholipid antibody (APLA)—to diagnose antibodies against the respective components of the body and useful for diagnosis of systemic lupus erythematosus and other similar diseases.

17. **Human leucocyte antigen (HLA) typing:** Human leucocyte antigens are a system of antigens which encode for proteins in the surface of cells for regulation of the immune system. The gene for HLA is in chromosome 6. They help to identify foreign substances and try to eliminate them. HLA typing is to find out the degree of matching between the donor and recipient before renal transplantation.

18. **MLC crossmatch:** It is a test done to rule out if the recipient has antibodies against the donor cells. The test is done before transplantation. It will not be possible to perform transplantation if the test is positive.

19. Cystatin C is a protein in the blood which is produced at a constant rate. Since it is filtered by the glomerulus and destroyed in the tubule constantly, the blood level remains constant in the range of 0.85 to 1.12 mg/L. It can be used as a reliable indicator of GFR. The level in blood rises if the filtration is affected.

20. Beta-2 microglobulin may also be used as a marker of glomerular filtration.

A few new markers like kidney injury molecule 1 (KIM-1), N-acetylglucosaminidase (NAG) and neutrophil gelatinase associated lipocalin (NGAL) have been identified and are useful markers of tubular damage.

More and more investigations are developed for studying renal diseases. All the above blood investigations need not be performed in all cases of renal failure. It is necessary to select the appropriate blood test so that a correct diagnosis can be made and treatment decided. Some of these tests have to be repeated for assessing the improvement or progress of the disease.

7

Importance of Imaging Urinary Tract

R Kasi Visweswaran, Satheesh Balakrishnan

X-rays were discovered more than 100 years back. This was followed by tomography, ultrasonography, Doppler studies, computerized axial tomography (CAT, scan) magnetic resonance imaging (MRI) and more recently, techniques like positron emission tomography (PET scan). Imaging of body parts to assess their structure and functions has become a very important part of investigations. When assessing the urinary tract any of the following investigations may be undertaken as indicated.

PLAIN X-RAYS ABDOMEN FOR KIDNEYS, URETERS AND BLADDER (X-RAY KUB)

This test helps to confirm

1. Adequate bowel preparations before taking contrast radiography
2. Identify radiopaque stones in the urinary system
3. Rule out bowel perforation
4. Identify radiopaque foreign bodies
5. Study gas shadows in intestinal obstruction
6. Look for 'air fluid' level

For a good X-ray KUB the patient is advised to use a laxative and gas absorbent (activates charcoal) for 2 days and report for X-ray on an empty stomach after evacuating the bowel in the morning. This reduces the bowel gas and gives a better visualization of the kidneys, ureter and bladder. If the X-ray examination is done later, even though the patient is starving, he may have swallowed air and the bowel may contain a lot of air and obscure the X-ray picture. If the preparation is adequate and X-ray settings are optimal, the shadow of the psoas muscle will be seen on either side of the spine as shown in Fig. 7.1. The renal outline and the outline of a distended bladder can also be seen.

INTRAVENOUS UROGRAM (IVU)/CT UROGRAM (CTU)

Intravenous urogram is done by preparing the patient as for X-ray KUB. The patient should be well hydrated. After test doses and confirming no allergic reaction, the contrast material is injected as a bolus intravenously. The contrast medium is filtered in the glomeruli, travels through the nephron, reaches the renal calyces and pelvis, travels along the ureter and accumulates in the bladder. Thereafter when the patient is asked to pass urine the dye is also divided with the urine. The X-rays are taken at 1, 5, 10, 20, and 30 minutes. The X-ray in 1st minute is called nephrogram and it helps us to see the kidneys clearly, measure its size, study the shape and look for scars. In the 5th minute X-ray, we will be able to see the dye in the minor and major calyces and renal pelvis. Normally compassion is applied at the level of umbilicus for the first 10 minutes. The X-ray taken at 10 minutes will therefore show the whole upper urinary tract on both sides. The X-ray taken at 20 minutes is without the compression. The passage of the dye to

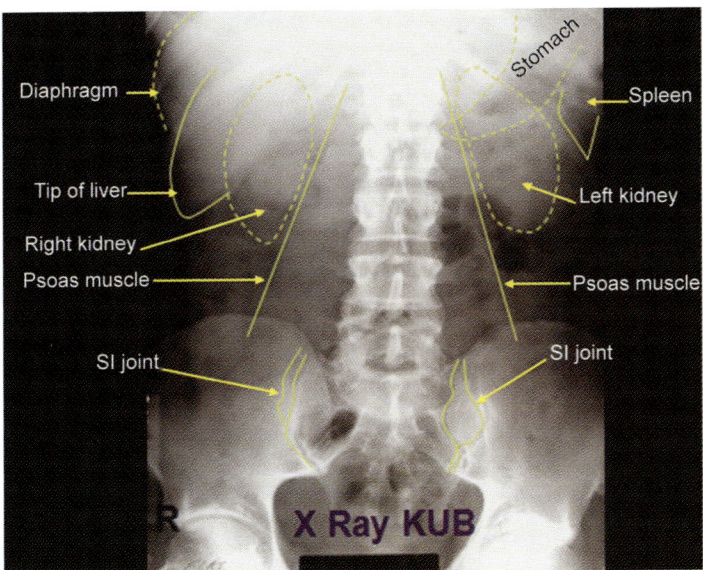

Fig. 7.1: Normal X-ray KUB showing important landmarks

the lower part of ureter and its entry to the bladder can be studied (Fig. 7.2). X-ray at 30 minutes focuses the full bladder for studying its details. Thereafter the patient is asked to empty the bladder by voiding and another X-ray taken to see if the bladder is empty, fully contracted. In some abnormal cases the dye may have gone up the ureter (vesicoureteric reflux) or filled up a pouch (vesical diverticulum) or the bladder may not have emptied itself completely.

When done with X-ray films, it is called intravenous urogram. When it is performed with a CT scan machine, it is called CT urogram. Since CT urogram provides greater information, it is now preferred over conventional IVU.

DIRECT PYELOGRAPHY

In direct pyelography the dilute contrast agent is injected directly into the renal calyx or ureter and X-rays taken to see the flow and presence of blocks. It also helps to see abnormalities in the mucosa, urinary leak, obstruction or diverticula. There are 2 types of direct pyelography. (Antegrade means following the same direction of

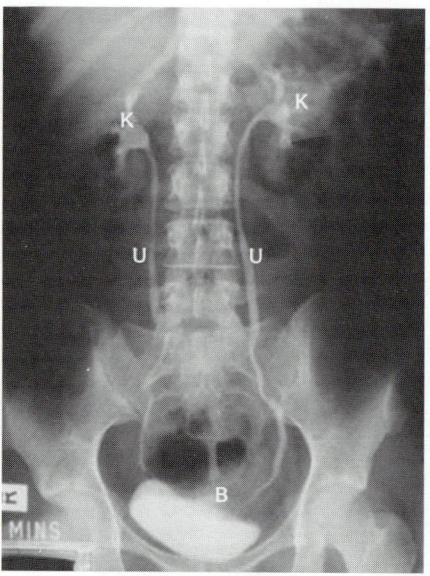

Fig. 7.2: Intravenous urogram showing kidneys (K), ureters (U) and bladder (B) filled with the contrast agent 20 minutes film of intravenous urogram

urine flow.) In antegrade pyelography the dilated renal calyx is punctured through the skin by a needle (under ultrasound guidance) and dye is injected into the collecting system and the X-ray is taken. This helps to study the flow of urine from the renal pelvis to bladder. (Retrograde means the dye is given in the direction opposite to the normal direction of flow of urine). In retrograde pyelogram the urologist introduces a catheter into the ureter through a cystoscope and injects the dye directly into the ureter. This helps to visualize the ureter and pelvicalyceal system clearly.

MICTURATING CYSTOURETHROGRAM

This study is done more commonly in children who have history of urinary tract infection. This test helps to rule out vesicoureteric reflux (VUR). In VUR, the urine from the bladder goes in retrograde (reverse) direction into the ureter when the bladder contrasts. Although the child may pass some urine, some urine from the bladder may travel even up the kidney and cause damage. For doing MCU, the child is positioned in the X-ray table, and a soft catheter is introduced into the bladder carefully taking all sterile precautions. The dilute contrast medium (dye) is introduced into the bladder. After removing the catheter, the child is asked to pass urine and X-rays are taken when the child is passing urine. Study of the X-ray will show if the bladder is normal in size, whether there are diverticula and whether urine is travelling in the reverse direction. Today, video cystogram and urodynamic studies are available to study the quantity, pressure of urine flow, urine flow rate, tone of muscles and coordinated action of muscles of bladder.

ULTRASONOGRAPHY AND DOPPLER STUDY

Ultrasonography is a simple non-invasive imaging modality. It can be repeated as need as it is non-invasive. It consists of a source for creating mechanical vibrational energy (ultrasound waves) and a receiver for the sound waves. Different tissues in the body modify and reflect the sound waves. These modified, reflected sound waves are recorded and displayed on a screen. It can be used to find out the presence, position, size, stone, obstruction cysts or tumors. It also helps to assess the size of stone, size or extent of dilatation of renal pelvis and calyx, size of cysts and residual urine after micturition. It helps to identify ectopic kidneys and other anomalies. With ultrasound guidance, we can do many procedures safely and successfully. Aspiration of fluid from body spaces, biopsy or FNAC from lesions in deeper tissue can be performed easily under ultrasound guidance. Most of these procedures were performed 'blindly' earlier and the complications were also more.

In Doppler test, the pattern of blood flow can be assessed. Significant obstruction can be identified. It can help to suspect renal artery stenosis, assess vascularity of tumors or check blood flow to transplanted kidneys. Power Doppler test helps to identify even minimal blood flow to a region.

RENAL ANGIOGRAPHY

Blood supply to kidney can be studied by injecting the dye directly into abdominal aorta and tracing its passage into the kidney. This called flush abdominal aortography. In this, we will be able to see the abdominal aorta and its major branches like celiac axis, superior mesenteric artery, both renal arteries, inferior mesenteric arteries and both external iliac arteries. After identifying the renal artery, it is possible to catheterise selectively one renal artery and inject the dye. This is called selective renal angiography. Abnormalities in the blood vessel such as narrowing (stenosis), aneurysm or arteriovenous malformation can be identified. Tumors of the kidney which are vascular will be seen clearly because there will be more dye in the tumor than the surrounding. Angiogram can be followed by procedures like renal angioplasty, stenting or embolisation as needed. Digital subtraction angiogram gives more clear picture after cancelling the bony parts in the X-ray. Angiography done with a CT machine helps to reconstruct 3D images of the part studied through computerized programs.

COMPUTERIZED AXIAL TOMOGRAPHY (CAT) SCAN

CAT scan or CT scan or X-ray CT is a combination of many X-ray images taken from different angles at the same time. These images are combined by the computer to provide cross-sectional images (Fig. 7.3). It will be possible to see the images of sections of the body at various levels. So the body parts can be studied in greater detail. Radiocontrast agents can be used to increase the visualization of vascular organs. From these data, the computer can reconstruct 3-dimensional reconstruction images which give life-like pictures.

Note: Aorta, both kidneys and stomach are clearly seen as white (the white color is due to the radiocontrast in the stomach and blood).

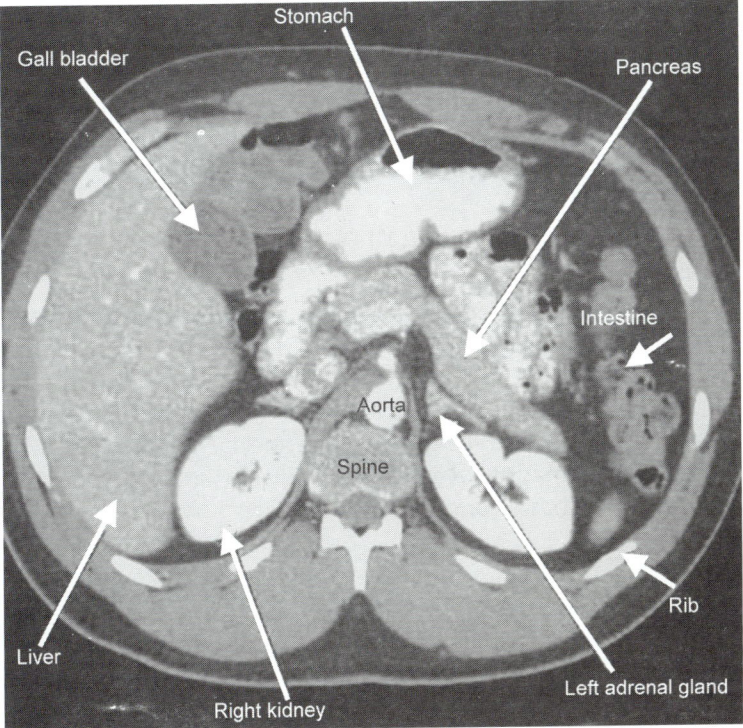

Fig. 7.3: CT scan of abdomen after oral and intravenous contrast administration

MAGNETIC RESONANCE IMAGING (MRI)

MRI is relatively less invasive investigation and helps in diagnosis. It uses powerful magnetic field and radiofrequency pulses. Those who have metallic implants, pacemakers or internal devices should not go near the machine when the machine is ON. Usually the procedure is done in a locked room where only the patient is kept. MRI is a painless procedure. The patient is usually warned that there will be loud and sudden thumping sounds and constant humming sound when the machine is functioning. All metallic objects, ornaments, clips, etc. should be removed before entering the room. Even heavy metallic objects can be attracted by the magnet and the object may 'fly' towards the magnet. The data obtained is fed into a computer which provides the images. However, the procedure does not involve ionizing radiations. Gadolinium is the contrast agent used to enhance MR images. Gadolinium will not be excreted and it will deposit in the body in patients with renal failure. Therefore, contrast MRI should be avoided in patients with renal failure. MRI is not as effective as CT in studying bones, calcification and calculi. In some situations like renal tumor, it helps to see the extent of involvement and vascular extension better than CT.

PET SCAN AND SINGLE-PHOTON EMISSION COMPUTED TOMOGRAPHY (SPECT)

These are newer modalities of nuclear imaging. PET scan uses a radionuclide tracer to produce a 3-dimensional image of the functioning part of the body. This can be combined with CT to give more information. SPECT scan is a type of nuclear imaging which uses radioactive substance and a special camera to produce 3-dimensional images which give information of not only the structure but also the function of body parts.

8

Importance of Radionuclide Studies

Manu G Krishnan, R Kasi Visweswaran

Nuclear imaging studies or nuclear scintigraphy, radiotracers or radiopharmaceuticals are used to study the structure and functions of the organs in the body. A radiopharmaceutical is a combination of a chemical compound to which a radioactive substance is tagged (attached). The chemical compounds and the radiotracers vary depending on the part or tissue of the body to be studied. When such a substance is administered, it localized in a tissue depending on the character of the chemical compound. A radioactive substance emits radiations in the form of alpha rays, beta rays and gamma rays. Gamma rays emitted by the radioactive substance is captured by a gamma camera and generates an image or graph. The study of the image or graph can give an idea about the position, size, structure and function of the tissue studied. For example, when iodine is administered, it is concentrated mainly in the thyroid gland. Radioactive iodine (^{131}I) is used to study the thyroid gland. The presence and distribution or the radiotracer in the body helps to assess its position, size, presence of 'hot' (overfunctioning), 'cold' (nonfunctioning areas) within the thyroid gland or presence of ectopic functioning tissue. In nephrology, nuclear imaging can be used to assess renal blood flow, glomerular filtration rate (GFR), renal transit time, obstruction to urinary tract and study the urinary bladder are used for diagnosis. Renal uptake can be calculated by the gamma camera during renography and is a good indicator for individual as well as overall kidney function. It is easy and non-invasive, and can give an idea about individual kidney function. It is less accurate compared to blood tests and clearance studies.

RENAL RADIOPHARMACEUTICALS USED IN NEPHROLOGY

Isotope scanning is a useful investigation for evaluation of kidneys and urinary tract. It provides information about blood flow to the kidneys, glomerular filtration, overall tubular function, drainage of urine from renal pelvis to bladder, presence of vesicoureteric reflux and relative functions of each kidney. It is also useful in the assessment of the transplanted kidney.

Table 8.1 summarises the main uses of isotope renography and the radiopharmaceutical used.

The most commonly employed scans are DTPA renogram and DMSA scan.

DTPA Renogram

99 m Tc DTPA is used for isotope renogram. When administered intravenously, it is filtered by the glomeruli and excreted in the urine. The passage of the radiotracer through the blood, kidney and urinary tract can be visualized in serial images. If the blood supply to one side is blocked, the radiotracer will not be seen on that side. If the renal artery is narrowed, the size of the kidney will be smaller and the appearance of the radiotracer will be delayed on that side. If 25 mg captopril is administered 1 hour before the scan, the function on the affected will be decrease further. This is called Captopril renogram and is done to confirm renal artery stenosis on one side. If the glomerular filtration (kidney function) is diminished, the radiotracer will not outline the kidney well. If the tubules are damaged, the tracer will remain in the kidney longer. If there is urinary obstruction, the tracer will remain in the collecting system longer. In pelviureteric junction obstruction, the tracer will remain in the dilated renal pelvis and will not drain into the bladder. To find out if the obstruction is significant or not, DTPA renogram with diuretic is performed. For this, the patient is hydrated well, given 20 mg frusemide intravenously just before injecting the tracer and scan performed. If the obstruction is significant, the tracer will remain in the renal pelvis, whereas if the obstruction is partial or dynamic, the tracer will be draining well after the diuretic. This is called diuretic. The DTPA renogram can also help to find out the contribution from each kidney to the overall kidney function.

DMSA Scan

Since DMSA remains in the renal parenchyma longer, it is useful to study the parenchyma for scars. DMSA can identify

Table 8.1: Uses of isotope renography and the radiopharmaceutical used

Function assessed	Abbreviation	Substance used	Radiotracer	Pharmaceutical	Remarks
Glomerular filtration rate	GFR	99m Tc-DTPA	Technetium	DTPA	Diethylene triamine penta-acetic acid (DTPA)
		51 Cr-EDTA	Chromium	EDTA	Ethylenediamine-tetra-acetic acid (EDTA)
Tubular secretion	ERPF	123I–	Iodine	Iodine	Iodine
		131I–OIH	Iodine	OIH	Orthoiodohippurate (OIH)
		99m Tc-MAG3 MAG3	Technetium	MAG3	Mercaptoacetyltriglycine (MAG3)
		99m Tc-EC	Technetium	EC	Ethylcysteine (EC)
Tubular retention	Imaging for cortical scars	99m Tc-DMSA	Technetium	DMSA	Dimercaptosuccinic acid
		99m Tc-GH	Technetium	GH	

Note:

1. 99m Tc-MAG3 is highly protein bound and is also cleared mainly by the proximal tubules. It will produce better scintigraphic images even in patients with impaired renal function.
2. 99m Tc-ethylenedicysteine (EC) is excellent radiopharmaceutical for renal studies.
3. 99m Tc-dimercaptosuccinic acid (DMSA) concentrates in the renal cortex and produces excellent cortical imaging.
4. 99m Tc-glucoheptonate (GH) is an agent that is filtered by the glomerulus and bound by the tubules. Hence, useful in assessing tubular function.
5. Progressive accumulation of OIH or 99m Tc-MAG3 in the parenchyma is a good prognostic feature in acute tubular necrosis.

non-functioning areas in parenchyma as photopenic areas (areas not having radioactive tracer in the parenchyma). Thus, it will help in diagnosing tumors, cysts, abscesses, or infarcts. In the case of infarcts, the photopenic areas are wedge shaped.

TRANSPLANTATION RENOGRAPHY

After renal transplantation, isotope scan can be done to visualize and confirm if renal perfusion is adequate and to visualize the urinary tract. Information about different surgical complications like arterial stenosis, venous and arterial thrombosis, infarction, bleeding, urinary obstruction or leakage can be obtained and diagnosed with appropriate tests.

Radionuclide scanning or isotope scanning is newer modality of investigation and has an important role in assessing kidneys and urinary tract.

9

Importance of Kidney Biopsy

R Kasi Visweswaran, Jose Paul

A renal biopsy is an invasive procedure wherein a piece of renal tissue is obtained from the kidney using a biopsy gun (Fig. 9.1). This is done under sonological guidance after confirming that both kidneys are present and there is no bleeding disorder. It is performed under local anesthesia in the side room or minor procedure room. There is no need for fasting but the patient should not have had a heavy meal during the past 3 hours.

PREBIOPSY PREPARATION

The procedure in most of the centers is done either as a day procedure, or as one requiring an overnight admission after the procedure. The patient and the relatives are counselled about the procedure, and an informed and written consent is taken.

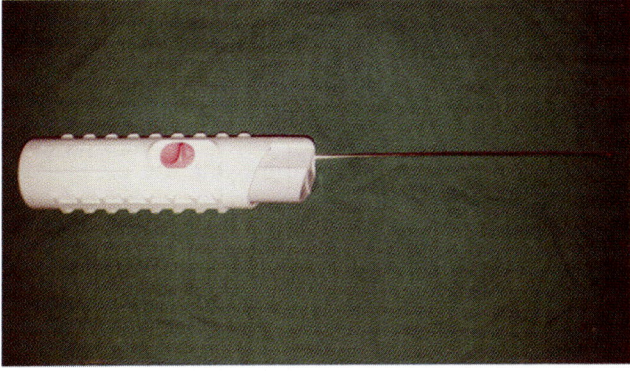

Fig. 9.1: Renal biopsy gun—note the long needle, spring loaded device (white) and the firing trigger (pink)

The hemogram, platelet count, renal function tests and the bleeding and coagulation parameters (prothrombin time/activated partial thromboplastin time) are assessed. Special care should be taken to review the medication history of the patient and to note whether the patient is on any antiplatelet drugs, which are stopped one week prior to the procedure. The site for the biopsy can be marked on the skin and the depth of the kidney from the skin assessed by ultrasonography. Realtime ultrasonography may also be used to guide the needle of the biopsy gun to the renal cortex. The patient is positioned in prone position and trained to hold the breath in inspiration for a few seconds. A sand bag or small pillow in the upper abdomen helps to support the kidney and enable easier biopsy. The lower pole of the left kidney is marked when the patient holds his breath in deep inspiration.

SETTING UP A TRAY FOR RENAL BIOPSY

The tray should contain

1. Sterile drapes
2. Sterile gloves
3. Sterile gauze pieces
4. Sterile cotton balls
5. 5 ml syringe with short and long needles for administration of local anesthetic
6. Renal biopsy gun
7. Strict sterile precautions are necessary during the procedure.

Biopsy Procedure

The procedure is done under ultrasound guidance. It is also possible to mark the site and depth of the kidney from skin by ultrasonography and do the biopsy later. The patient is made to lie prone on the bed with small pillow in the upper abdomen. The skin is cleaned with antiseptic solution and the site is draped with sterile 'hole towel'. The skin, subcutaneous tissue and deeper structures including the peri-renal fascia are infiltrated with xylocaine for local anesthesia. A small stab incision is made on the marked skin site with a number 11 surgical blade to enable easy introduction of the needle of the biopsy gun through the skin. The patient must be told that there will be snapping sound heard and felt when the gun is activated. A guiding needle often, a lumbar puncture needle is introduced to the appropriate depth. The needle will be seen to move with respiration if the tip is in the kidney. The needle of the biopsy gun is then introduced through the incision till the marked depth while the patient holds the breath in deep inspiration. The biopsy gun is fired and withdrawn. The sample is taken from the slot in the inner needle of the gun and placed in the appropriate bottles. The incision site is covered with gauze piece and dressings applied. It is advisable to apply external pressure with the palm of the hand over the biopsy site with a view to prevent the development of large perirenal hematoma.

The patient is asked to lie prone for an hour and to take complete bed rest for 24 hours. The pulse and blood pressure is monitored on any half hourly basis for two hours followed later by hourly monitoring. The patient is also instructed to collect three consecutive urine samples and advised to inform the nursing staff if there is hematuria.

Indications for Renal Biopsy

1. Diagnosing glomerular diseases including nephrotic syndrome in adults
2. Unexplained acute renal failure
3. Postrenal transplant patient—diagnosis of various types of rejection.
4. To diagnose, assess prognosis and plan treatment—SLE with lupus nephritis, vasculitis with renal involvement.
5. Unexplained chronic kidney disease

Contraindications for Renal Biopsy

There are absolute and relative contraindications.

Absolute Contraindications

1. Bleeding disorders
2. Renal neoplasm

Relative Contraindications

1. Solitary kidney (renal transplant is an exception)
2. Uncontrolled blood pressure
3. Active upper urinary tract infection/abscess
4. Severe uremia (increased risk of bleeding)
5. Ectopic kidney
6. Skin infection at the site of biopsy.

Postbiopsy Care

In most centers, biopsy is done as a day procedure/outpatient. It is advisable to observe the patient for 24 hours for bleeding or hypotension. Bed rest is advised for 24 hours. Charting of pulse rate, blood pressure and observing urine samples for gross hematuria are done in the hospital.

Complications of Renal Biopsy

The following complications, renal biopsy has markedly reduced after improvements in the imaging modalities and with the introduction of the biopsy gun.

The common complications which are encountered are:

1. **Pain:** Usually dull aching at the site of renal biopsy which responds to simple analgesics. A persistent severe pain should suggest the possibility of bleeding around the kidney (perinephric or perirenal hematoma). An ultrasonogram helps to rule out perinephric hematoma.

2. **Hemorrhage:** In addition to perirenal hematoma, bleeding can happen into the renal pelvis which results in passing large quantities of blood or even clots in urine after biopsy (gross hematuria). Usually this responds to strict bed rest and blood transfusions, if necessary. If persistent bleeding occurs, renal angiography and embolisation of the bleeding artery will be necessary.

3. **Other complications:** Renal arteriovenous fistula may form after a few weeks if the needle has injured an artery and vein inside the kidney.

4. **Accidental perforation of other organs:** Liver, spleen, lungs may occur. Rarely, hypotension, massive hemorrhage or even death may occur.

PROCESSING AND DESPATCH OF SAMPLE TO THE LABORATORY

Usually, one or two bits are taken through the biopsy gun. The specimen is divided into three samples:

1. One in formaldehyde solution for light microscopy
2. One in normal saline or transport medium for immuno-fluorescence study
3. One sample stored in glutaraldehyde for electron microscopy study.

Ideally the biopsy sample should contain at least 10–15 glomeruli for making a useful histological diagnosis. The biopsy is processed for histopathologic examination by regular special stains as necessary. Immunofluorescence microscopy or immunoperoxidase stains are done to study the immune deposits in the kidney. Although electron microscopy is not necessary in all cases, it gives additional information about the ultrastructure of the kidney cells.

10

Signs and Symptoms of Renal Diseases

Reena Thomas

Renal disease can vary from asymptomatic and mild problems like postural proteinuria to severe renal failure. It is important to determine whether this is a relatively harmless problem or a forerunner of a serious renal disease. Signs and symptoms of kidney disease are also often nonspecific. Because the kidneys are highly adaptable and able to compensate for lost function, signs and symptoms may not appear until irreversible advanced damage has occurred.

A patient with disease of the kidneys or urinary system may seek medical attention with symptoms and signs of renal disease or with no symptoms referable to renal disease or abnormality detected on urine examination, routine blood tests or imaging techniques. Such abnormalities could be noted while investigating for unrelated diseases. Renal diseases can also present as a complication of a multi-system illness like diabetes mellitus, hypertension or vasculitis.

PRESENTING SYMPTOMS OF RENAL DISEASES

Some of the common symptoms with which renal disease may present are summarized here. (Please see corresponding chapters for details.)

Changes in Urine Volume

Oliguria

Decreased urine output or oliguria is a sign of impaired renal function. Oliguria is defined as a urine output that is less than 1 ml/kg/h in infants, less than 0.5 ml/kg/h in children, and less than 400 ml daily in adults. It is a symptom which helps the doctors to suspect renal disease.

Anuria

It is a condition where the patient passes less than 100 ml of urine in a day. Anuria is often caused by failure in the function of kidneys. It may also occur because of obstruction to the flow of urine. If the patient does not pass even a drop of urine, total obstruction should be suspected.

Polyuria

It is defined as excessive or abnormally large production or passage of urine (greater than 3000 ml over 24 hours in adults).

Nocturia

Its a common symptom of renal failure. It is defined as need to wake up at night to void urine. This may occur when kidneys are chronically damaged and the power to concentrate the urine during sleep is lost. In normal persons, the urine formed during sleeping hours is less than when the person is awake.

Changes in Urine Color

- *Red/pink color:* Blood, hemoglobin, menstrual contamination, beet-root, drugs—pyridium, rifampicin, warfarin.
- *Deep yellow color:* Jaundice
- *Cola color:* Hematuria (acute nephritis), hemoglobinuria, myoglobinuria.
- *Brown/black:* Phenylketonuria, drugs—nitrofurantoin, metro-nidazole, iron sorbitol.

Changes in Composition of Urine

Microalbuminuria

Moderately increased albuminuria: The daily albumin excretion in a normal person is <30 mg. Microalbuminuria is now referred to as moderately increased albuminuria. The urinary albumin excretion in this condition is between 30 and 300 mg of albumin daily (20–200 µg/minute). It can be detected by special albumin-specific urine dipstix test or radioimmunoassay. It is an important prognostic marker for kidney disease in diabetes mellitus, cardiovascular disease and hypertension.

Proteinuria

Normal urinary protein excretion is < 150 mg/24 hour. If more than 500 mg/day, it can be detected by simple laboratory tests. It causes the urine to become frothy or foamy. Proteinuria can be divided into three categories: Transient (intermittent), orthostatic (only in erect position) and persistent (always present). Proteinuria may be of different types and severity. It is classified on the basis of the quantity of protein in urine as nephrotic or non-nephrotic, the type of protein as albuminuria or low molecular weight proteinuria, or the underlying pathological damage as glomerular, non-glomerular, tubular and overflow proteinuria.

Chart below shows common types of proteinuria, their mechanism and type of damage.

Glomerular	Increased protein leak from glomerulus	Primary or secondary glomerular disease
Tubular	Decreased reabsorption of proteins by tubules	Tubular or interstitial disease
Overflow	Increased blood level and overflow of low-molecular-weight proteins	Monoclonal gammopathy, leukemia

Hematuria

It is defined as three or more red blood cells per high-power microscopic field in a centrifuged urinary sediment. The urine color may be normal, or smoky, cola colored, pink or red. It can be gross or only microscopic hematuria. If blood is seen in beginning of micturation, it suggests bleeding from the urethra, or bladder neck or prostate. Uniform bleeding may be due to renal causes or due to systemic causes of bleeding. Terminal bleeding may be indicating bleeding from the bladder. Gross hematuria with blood clots may occur with stones or tumors.

Casts

Presence of casts in urine suggests diseases of renal parenchyma.

Symptoms in Renal Diseases

The symptoms due to renal diseases are extremely variable. Patient may present to any specialty with corresponding symptoms—hematology department for anemia or bleeding tendency, infertility clinic, gynecologist for amenorrhea, orthopedic surgeon for bone pain or deformities, ophthalmologist for dimness of vision due to hypertensive retinopathy, neurologist for headache, gastroenterologist for GI symptoms, dermatologist for dry skin or itching, cardiologist for dyspnea and chest pain or pulmonologist for dyspnea and rapid breathing. Early diagnosis can be made only if renal disease is suspected in the above situations. Some symptoms will point directly to kidney disease. They are as follows.

Edema

Accumulation of excessive fluid in the interstitial compartment of the body gives rise to edema. Kidney diseases are associated with inability to excrete water from the body. Edema is an important sign of renal disease. Edema may also occur due to congestive heart failure, cirrhosis of liver, nutritional deficiency, or as side-effect of drugs (nonsteroidal anti-inflammatory drugs and some blood pressure medications). Common kidney diseases causing edema are nephrotic syndrome, acute nephritis, chronic renal failure and acute kidney injury. The edema usually occurs around the eyelids and later become generalized.

Hypertension

Hypertension is a very common manifestation of kidney diseases. Kidney diseases can be the cause of hypertension and hypertension can cause worsening of kidney disease. When children or young persons develop kidney disease, kidney disease should be suspected.

Pain

The pain due to diseases of kidney or urinary tract is the characteristic of renal diseases. There are pain sensitive nerve fibers only in the renal capsule or 'collecting system' (renal calyces, pelvis, ureter, bladder and urethra). When there is swelling of the kidney and stretching of renal capsule occurs, the patient experiences dull aching pain in the loin area. Renal colic is due to stone in the kidney or upper urinary tract. The pain is sharp and severe and radiates from the loin to the inguinal region, inner side of upper thigh, scrotum or vulva. The pain due to renal colic does not radiate to lateral aspect of thigh. The patient is often in distress and does not find comfort in any position. On the right side, the pain may resemble appendicitis. In contrast to renal colic, the patient with appendicitis prefers not to move from his comfortable position because any movement will worsen the pain. Bladder tumors or stone cause pain in the suprapubic region.

Abnormalities in Micturition

The act of passing urine (urination) is also called micturition. Normal persons are able to pass urine without any pain and can control the micturition. The common abnormalities and corresponding terms used are given below:

a. **Burning micturition:** Any infection in the urinary tract may result in burning sensation during micturition.

b. **Dysuria:** The term used for pain during micturition.

c. **Strangury:** The patient has a painful desire to pass urine even though the bladder is empty.

d. **Frequency of micturition:** The patient has to go for urination more frequently. (This can be due to reduced bladder capacity or inflammation in the bladder or urethra.)

e. **Hesitancy:** A condition where the patient will have difficulty in starting micturition. (This occurs usually in older men with prostatic enlargement.)

f. **Precipitancy:** It is the term used when the patient is forced to pass urine as soon as he feels the bladder sensation.

g. **Incontinence:** When the patient passes urine without control, the condition is called incontinence. There are many types of incontinence.

   i. *Continuous dribbling incontinence:* When there is continuous leakage of urine. (It may occur when there is a fistula between ureter or bladder and vagina.)

   ii. *Stress incontinence:* When the patient passes urine without control while coughing or laughing.

   iii. *Urge incontinence:* When the patient passes urine without control as soon as he feels bladder sensation.

   iv. *Postvoid dribbling:* When the patient passed some urine after completing the act of urination.

   v. *Overflow incontinence:* When the bladder is full, leak of urine may occur without the control of patient. (This can occur in neurological diseases where the control of micturition is lost.) This is also called 'retention with overflow'.

ABDOMINAL MASS

When the kidney is enlarged, it can be felt by palpation of abdomen. The procedure for palpating the kidney through the abdominal wall is called bimanual palpation. Cystic diseases of the kidney are a group of conditions where many cysts develop in one or both kidneys causing irregular enlargement. Autosomal dominant polycystic kidney disease (ADPKD) is a common disease with palpable kidneys due to many cysts in both kidneys. This is the commonest cause for enlarged kidneys. Other causes are tumors of the kidney, obstruction, abscess or injury (trauma).

UREMIC MANIFESTATIONS

As mentioned earlier, symptoms and signs (manifestations) due to uremia can be highly variable. The patient may have no symptoms at all till the renal function is less than GFR <30 ml/min (stage 4 of CKD). The symptoms in stages 4 and 5 are:

a. **Hypertension:** May be related to fluid and salt retention or due to renin release from the diseased kidney.

b. **Cardiovascular:** Cardiac muscle dysfunction, cardiac failure, uremic pericarditis, atherosclerosis and ischemic heart disease.

c. **Gastrointestinal:** Anorexia, nausea, vomiting, diarrhea, abdominal distension, and smell of ammonia in breath (uremic fetor).

d. **Neurological:** Numbness, 'restless leg' syndrome, peripheral neuropathy, bladder dysfunction, flapping tremor and myoclonus.

e. **Psychiatric:** Dementia, delirium, depression, agitation, coma or convulsions (due to electrolyte abnormalities).

f. **Respiratory:** Pleurisy, Kussmaul's breathing (deep sighing respiration due to metabolic acidosis) or pulmonary edema.

g. **Skin and nails:** Sallow complexion (pallor and pale yellow skin color due to deposition of a pigment called 'urochrome'), dry scaly skin, scratch marks, 'prurigo nodularis' (also called Kyrle's disease), calcification in skin, bleeding into skin, red eye, nail changes (pitting, 'half and half nails', or skin infections).

h. **Immune system:** Immunosuppressed state (prone for infections)

i. **Skeletal system:** Bone pain due to renal osteodystrophy, bone deformities in children due to rickets, features of hyperparathyroidism and vitamin D deficiency.

j. **Anemia:** Due to iron and erythropoietin deficiency.

k. **Reproductive system:** Amenorrhea, infertility, gynecomastia, gonadal dysfunction and impotence.

CLINICAL SYNDROMES IN NEPHROLOGY

When a patient presents with suspected renal disease, history, physical examination and preliminary investigations are done first. On the basis of the results, the disease is classified and a provisional diagnosis is made. There are 10 important syndromes in nephrology. Most patients will fit into one of the syndromes. Once the syndrome is identified correctly, the correct diagnosis can be made by further analysis and investigations. The 10 syndromes are:

1. Acute nephritic syndrome
2. Nephrotic syndrome
3. Acute kidney injury
4. Chronic kidney disease
5. Urinary tract infections
6. Urinary tract obstructions
7. Renal tubular defects
   (Structural tubular defects are mainly the various types of renal cysts or tumors and functional tubular defects are mainly renal tubular acidosis and acute kidney injury)
8. Urolithiasis (stone diseases)
9. Hypertension
10. Asymptomatic urinary abnormalities.

Each condition is explained in detail in separate chapters.

11

Acute Nephritic Syndrome

Reena Thomas

An acute nephritic syndrome is a group of renal disease that has a common presentation, namely:

1. Sudden onset of cola or dark colored urine. The urine examination often shows proteinuria and urine sediment with RBCs, granular and RBC casts. This is called nephritic or active urine sediment.
2. Sudden onset of facial (periorbital) puffiness which may progress to generalized edema.
3. Hypertension.

The clinical features are due to damage to glomeruli. The basement membrane, capillary endothelium and epithelium are damaged. The damaged glomerulus allows the escape of RBCs and proteins in urine. The white blood cells crowding the filtering glomerular tufts decrease the GFR. Decreased GFR leads to salt and fluid retension, edema, elevated jugular venous pressure, dyspnea, and hypertension. Sometimes sudden increase in blood pressure occurs with development of convulsions (fits). This is called hypertensive encephalopathy. A number of renal and systemic diseases can present with such nephritic presentation and we have to make a diagnosis depending on the history and clinical tests.

CAUSES (ETIOLOGY) OF ACUTE NEPHRITIC SYNDROME

Infections

1. Poststreptococcal acute glomerulonephritis (PSAGN).
2. Other bacterial infections:
   - Staphylococci
   - *Salmonella typhi*

- Brucella
- *Treponema pallidum*
3. Viruses:
   - Cytomegalovirus (CMV)
   - Epstein-Barr virus (EBV)
   - Hepatitis B virus
   - Rubella virus
   - Mumps virus
4. Rickettsial infections—scrub typhus
5. Parasitic infection—malarial parasite (*Plasmodium falciparum* and *P. malariae*)
6. Fungi: *Toxoplasma gondii*.

Noninfective Causes

Primary renal diseases:
- Membranoproliferative glomerulonephritis (MPGN)
- IgA nephropathy (nephropathy due to immunoglobulin A)
- Rapidly progressive glomerulonephritis (RPGN)

Multisystem Disease

- Vasculitis:
  - Wegener's granulomatosis
  - Polyarteritis nodosa (PAN)
  - Henoch-Schönlein purpura (HSP)
  - Collagen vascular disease, e.g. systemic lupus erythematosus (SLE)
  - Goodpasture syndrome

Thus, any patient coming with nephritic presentation could be suffering from any of the above diseases. A detailed history, clinical examination and appropriate investigations are necessary to come to a correct diagnosis and offer treatment.

POSTSTREPTOCOCCAL ACUTE GLOMERULONEPHRITIS

The disease is more common in young children living in overcrowded areas but is also seen in older people. Often, this is preceded by evidence of streptococcal infection. Symptoms of acute nephritis may start 7–10 days after streptoccoal pharyngitis and 2–3 weeks following skin infection (pyoderma). Some strains of beta hemolytic streptococci cause nephritis. They are called nephritogenic strains. Group A, beta hemolytic streptococci have a number of strains but not all cause nephritis. The nephrotogenic strains, M type strain, types 1, 2, 4, and 12 causing throat infection and types 25, 47, 49 producing skin infection are followed by PSAGN.

PSAGN is the prototype of acute nephritic syndrome. When infection occurs, the body produces antibodies against the streptococcal antigen. The antibody level in the blood increases during the first few weeks. The antigens and antibodies combine to form immune complexes. About 2–3 weeks after the infection occurs, there will be sufficient antibodies to form immune complexes and they get deposited in the glomeruli. This results in invasion of the glomerulus by white cells, activation of complement system, cytokines and other mediators of inflammation. Thus acute nephritic syndrome is an immunologically mediated acute inflammation of the glomeruli. The streptococcal agent may also directly damage the glomerular basement membrane.

It may occur as endemic in overcrowded areas. In many cases, the illness may be subclinical or mild nephritis. Others will have the typical clinical course while a few may have a complicated course. The complications are more common in adults than children. The important complications are hypertensive encephalopathy, acute renal failure, hyperkalemia and fluid overload.

The clinical presentation is extremely variable. It may be asymptomatic subclinical nephritis which may go unnoticed. It may present as microscopic hematuria, typical acute nephritic syndrome as described above, nephrotic syndrome, severe hypertension or acute renal failure. On examination, there may be scars of recent skin infection, facial puffiness, generalized edema, hypertension, features of circulatory overload, raised JVP, dyspnea, basal crepitation in lungs. The disease has a self-limiting course. After about a week or 10 days, the urine output increases, hematuria clears and complete recovery occurs. A few patients may develop hypertensive encephalopathy, hyperkalemia, or renal failure.

Urine examination will show proteinuria which may be minimal. The 24-hour urine protein is often less than <2 gm. Urine microscopy will show RBC, RBC casts and granular casts. The RBCs may not be having normal shape and the morphology may be abnormal (dysmorphic) if examined under phase contrast microscope.

Examination of the blood may show transient elevation of serum creatinine, blood urea or potassium. Serum complement levels are low (hypocomplementemia) during the first 1–2 weeks. The following serological tests help to confirm infection with streptococci.

    a. Anti-streptolysin (ASO)—commonly done—ASO titers > 200 units are significant.
    b. Anti-hyaluronidase (AH ase)
    c. Anti-streptokinase (ASKase)
    d. Anti-nicotinamide-adenine dinucleotidase (anti-NAD)
    e. Anti-DNAse B antibodies

Kidney biopsy is usually not necessary for children with acute nephritis. It is recommended for all adults with acute nephritic syndrome. In children it is indicated under the following conditions:

    a. Persistently low C3 levels beyond six weeks (suggest a diagnosis of membranoproliferative glomerulonephritis).
    b. Recurrent episodes of hematuria occurring with infections (suggestive of IgA nephropathy)
    c. A progressive increase in serum creatinine (rapidly progressive glomerulonephritis)

The kidneys are enlarged and the kidney biopsy may show swelling of the glomeruli with proliferation of cells in the glomerulus and presence of polymorphonuclear cells (neutrophils). This histological picture is called diffuse endocapillary proliferative glomerulonephritis (Fig. 11.1). By immunofluorescence microscopy and electron microscopy, it will be possible to see the immune complexes deposited in the glomeruli.

DIFFERENTIAL DIAGNOSIS

If the patient presents with typical features, the diagnosis acute nephritic syndrome is easy. To differentiate PSAGN from other causes, further investigations are necessary. If there is an evidence of recent infection with group A beta-hemolytic streptococci, and the nephritis resolves within two to three weeks of presentation, the diagnosis of uncomplicated PSAGN can be confirmed. Renal biopsy helps to differentiate between various types of acute nephritic syndrome.

• *Membranoproliferative glomerulonephritis (MPGN):* Patients with MPGN may present initially like PSAGN with hematuria, hypertension, proteinuria, and hypocomplementemia following

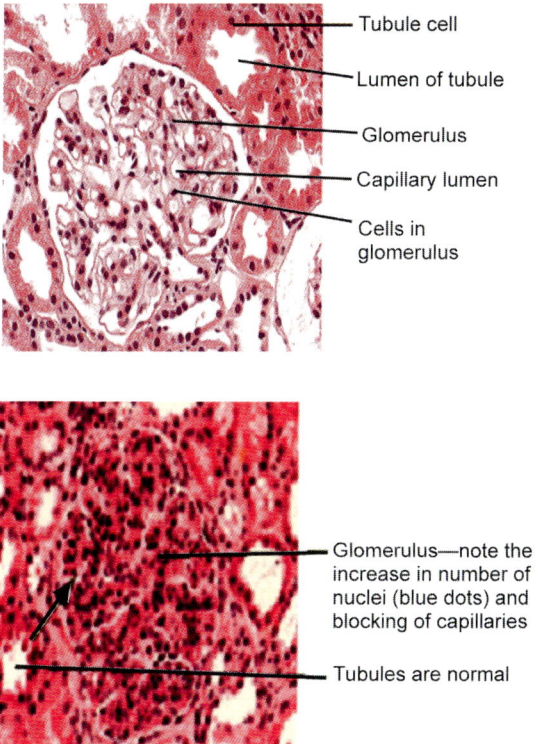

Tubule cell

Lumen of tubule

Glomerulus

Capillary lumen

Cells in glomerulus

Glomerulus—note the increase in number of nuclei (blue dots) and blocking of capillaries

Tubules are normal

Fig. 11.1: Normal glomerulus showing the normal cells and capillary loops (upper panel). On the lower panel, numerous cells (blue dots are nuclei) are seen inside the glomerulus and capillaries are blocked by the swelling due to cells (no blood flow through the capillaries)

an upper respiratory infection. However, patients with MPGN continue to have persistent features of nephritis, low levels of serum complement (hypocomplementemia) and significant proteinuria persisting for more than four to six weeks. They may also have progressive renal failure.

- *IgA nephropathy:* Patients with IgA nephropathy often present after an upper respiratory infection, similar to the presentation of patients with PSAGN. A shorter time interval between the upper respiratory infection and hematuria is present in IgA nephropathy. The interval is usually less than 5 days, whereas it is more than 10 days in PSAGN. Prior episodes of gross hematuria may also be present. Recurrence of hematuria is rare if PSAGN has recovered completely.

- *Secondary glomerulonephritis:* Systemic lupus erythematosus (SLE) and Henoch-Schönlein purpura (HSP) share similar features to PSGN. Both these conditions have other manifestation.

- Both hepatitis B and endocarditis-associated glomerulonephritis share common features with PSGN and also have deficiency of C3 and C4.

- *Postinfectious GN due to other microbial agents:* Acute nephritis due to viral and other bacterial agents occur. Although their clinical presentation is similar to PSAGN, there will be no evidence of streptococcal infection.

MANAGEMENT

Management of PSGN is supportive as the disease is usually self limiting. A course of antibiotics is given if active infection is present. Often the illness occurs after the infection is controlled. Daily weight chart and strict fluid balance chart should be maintained. Fluid intake should be monitored and maintained to 400 ml (insensible loss on a moderately warm day) plus the amount equal to the previous day's output. This is in order to prevent fluid overload. Salt and fluid restriction are necessary if there is evidence of fluid overload. Diuretic like frusemide may be used if there is oliguria or gross edema. Strenuous physical activity should be avoided. Blood pressure is monitored every 4 hours and drug treatment started if BP increases. Hypertension should be controlled by appropriate antihypertensive drugs. If there is acute renal failure, protein and potassium restriction should be enforced. The serum K levels should be monitored. Dialysis may be required if there is acute renal failure, severe fluid overload or hyperkalemia.

Complications: Most patients recover spontaneously and with supportive measures. Congestive cardiac failure and hypertensive encephalopathy can occur. Rarely a nephrotic syndrome and ARF can occur. *Crescentic glomerulonephritis* is suspected if the symptoms persist and the serum creatinine level increases progressively. In such cases, early renal biopsy is done so that specific treatment can be initiated early. Urinary abnormalities like microscopic hematuria and proteinuria can persists for 3–6 weeks. If proteinuria or microscopic hematuria persist for more than 3 months, it may be necessary to do a biopsy even though the renal functions are normal.

Other Infective Causes of Acute Glomerulonephritis

The salient features of other organisms causing postinfectious glomerulonephritis are:

a. Shunt nephritis occurs due to staphalococci in patient with ventriculo-atrial shunt.
b. Infective endocarditis can also be a cause of glomerulonephritis.
c. Membranoproliferative glomerulonephritis occurs following infection by hepatitis B, hepatitis C or HIV.
d. Malarial parasite—*Plasmodium falciparum* and malaria can cause proliferative glomerulonephritis.
e. Schistosomiasis is also associated with nephritis.

Primary Renal Diseases Causing an Acute Nephritis

Membranoproliferative Glomerulonephritis (MPGN)

It is a type of nephrotic syndrome. The onset of the illness may be like acute nephritic syndrome associated with nephrotic range proteinuria. This is called nephritic-nephrotic onset. MPGN can be primary or idiopathy and secondary. Patients have proteinuria, hypertension, hematuria, and renal failure. The serum complement is often low. Renal biopsy shows the characteristic findings. MPGN can be idiopathic or secondary. Secondary MPGN may follow infections like Hepatitis B, C, infective endocarditis, shunt nephritis, malaria, or disease like Sjögren's syndrome, scleroderma, sarcoidosis or malignancies like leukemia, lymphoma and carcinoma.

IgA Nephropathy

This is the commonest cause for acute nephritis. It causes recurrent episodes of hematuria, microscopic or macroscopic. The episodes occur within 5 days after an upper respiratory infection. IgA is again an immune complex mediated disorder with deposits of IgA predominantly in the mesangium of the glomerulus. IgA nephropathy occurs due to an immune response to some foreign antigen or as a result of autoimmunity against the mesangial antigens. It can either be a primary disease or secondary to systemic disease like alcoholic liver disease, celiac and Crohn's diseases, psoriasis, ankylosing spondylitis, Hansen's disease or HIV.

Hereditary Nephritis (or Alport Syndrome)

It is an inherited disorder affecting all basement membranes of the body including the glomerular basement membrane. It is often associated with sensorineural hearing loss and ocular abnormalities like myopia. The high myopia is due to lenticonus. Alport syndrome is due to mutations of genes contolling type IV collagen proteins. This should be suspected in patients with family history of renal failure, eye and ear abnormalities having a history of repeated episodes of hematuria.

Approach to a patient presenting with acute nephritic syndrome is summarized below.

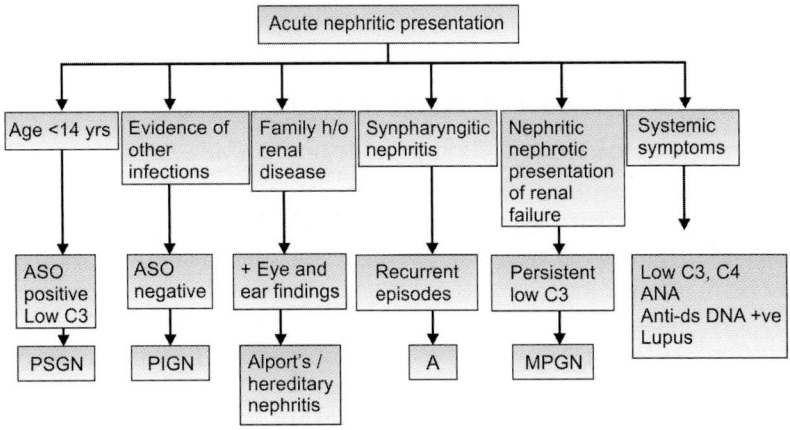

12

Nephrotic Syndrome

R Kasi Visweswaran

INTRODUCTION

Nephrotic syndrome is common in children and adults. Nephrotic syndrome can be defined as a condition characterised by proteinuria (>3.5 gm/day) which is often associated with hypoalbuminemia, edema and hyperlipidemia. The first event which occurs in nephrotic syndrome is excretion in urine of large quantities of protein and is due to damage to the glomerular capillary filtering mechanism (Fig. 12.1). If urine contains more than 2.0 gm of protein per square meter body surface area or 3.5 gm in 24 hours in adults,

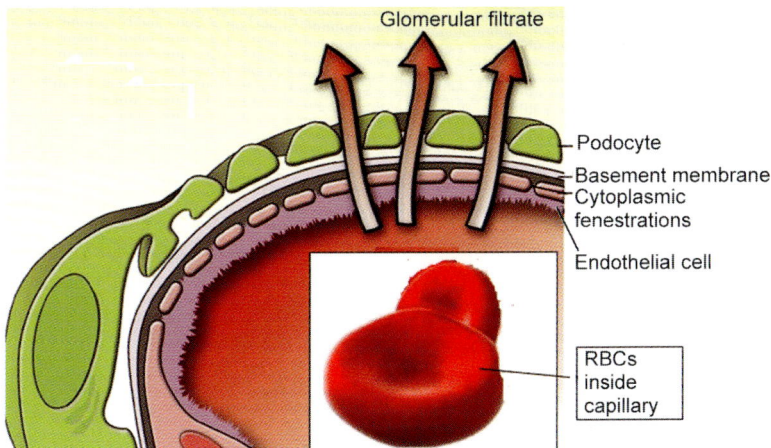

Fig. 12.1: Glomerular capillary filter

Figure 12.1 shows the 3 layers of the capillary endothelial filter: Endothelial cells with fenestrations, basement membrane and visceral epithelial cell (podocytes).

the condition is called nephrotic syndrome. The lost protein is mainly albumin and occurs due to damage to the glomerular capillary filter. As a result of loss of proteins from the body the patient may develop hypoalbuminemia. When the level of albumin decreases in blood, the fluid that moves out of the blood stream at the arterial end of the capillary cannot return to the blood. The fluid thus accumulates in the extracellular fluid compartment. Adequate level of albumin in blood is necessary for balancing the starling forces and causing movement of fluid to move from extracellular to intravascular compartment in the capillary. The patient develops edema which may appear as puffiness of eyelids on getting up in the morning. Later, in the day, it may appear as swelling of the ankles. In later stages the edema becomes generalized with development of ascites, pleural effusion and even pericardial effusion (anasarca). The liver tries to produce more albumin. The synthesis of albumin and lipoproteins in the liver are somewhat linked. Therefore, the liver produces more lipids like cholesterol. Because of this, the patients develop hyper-lipidemia (high levels of cholesterol and lipoproteins). The blood contains factors favoring clotting (procoagulant factors) and those which prevent clotting (anticoagulant factors). Balance between these factors prevent clotting of blood in the blood stream. These factors are also protein in nature. An important anticoagulant factor called Antithrombin 3 is excreted in these patients with gross proteinuria. Because of the loss of the anticoagulant factor, the pro coagulant factors cause clotting of blood within the blood stream (vascular thrombosis). The thrombosis can occur in the venous system or even within the arteries. Other proteins like thyroid binding globulin, vitamin D binding protein immunoglobulins and complement are also lost in urine resulting in hypothyroidism, vitamin D deficiency, and easy susceptibility to infection. The causes can be broadly classified as primary (idipopathic), where there is no specific cause, or secondary, where the nephrotic syndrome occurs due to a disease in other organs.

COMMON CAUSES

Common causes of nephrotic syndrome:

Primary Nephrotic Syndrome

1. Minimal change disease
2. Membranous nephropathy

3. Focal segmental glomerulosclerosis
4. Mesangioproliferative glomerulonephritis
5. Membranoproliferative glomerulonephritis
6. IgA nephropathy

Secondary Causes of Nephrotic Syndrome

1 Multisystem diseases
   a. Systemic lupus erythematosus
   b. Amyloidosis
   c. Sarcoidosis
   d. Other connective tissue disorders
2. Tumors
   a. Lung cancer
   b. Colon cancer
   c. Stomach cancer
   d. Breast cancer
   e. Lymphoma/leukemia
3. Infections
   a. HIV
   b. Hepatitis B
   c. Hepatitis C
   d. *Plasmodium malariae infection*
   e. Secondary syphilis
4. Drugs
   a. Penicillamine
   b. Gold
   c. Captopril
   d. Mercury
5. Metabolic diseases
   a. Diabetes mellitus
6. Miscellaneous
   a. Pre-eclampsia
   b. Vesicoureteric reflux
   c. Congenital nephrotic syndrome
   d. Insect bites.

Primary nephrotic syndrome is more common in children (90%) but in adults it is only (50%). If nephrotic syndrome occurs in a child before 1 year, it is likely to be congenital nephrotic syndrome.

CLINICAL FEATURES

The onset of the illness may be gradual and the patient may notice minimal puffiness of face on getting up in the morning which disappears after a few hours. Thereafter, the patient may notice swelling of the ankle region which may become generalized. In the simplest form of nephrotic syndrome like minimal change disease, there may not be any other findings on clinical examination. The urine examination will show proteinuria, the serum albumin level is often low and cholesterol level high. In other types of nephrotic syndrome, hypertension, microscopic hematuria (blood in urine test or RBCs in the urine by microscopy), renal failure may be present depending on the type of disease. In secondary nephrotic syndrome, clinical features of the main disease will be present. Primary symptoms include anorexia, malaise and frothy urine (caused by high concentrations of protein). Fluid retention may cause dyspnea due to pleural effusion, abdominal distension due to ascites, arthralgia, peripheral edema and ascites. Edema may obscure signs of muscle wasting. Parallel white lines in fingernail beds called Muehrcke lines may be seen. Other symptoms and signs attributable to the complications may be seen.

Diagnosis

The diagnosis can be made clinically by noting the distribution and character of the edema, by measuring 24-hour urine protein excretion and checking blood for hypoalbuminemia and hyperlipidemia. In primary nephrotic syndromes other than minimal change disease, there may variable degrees of hypertension, microscopic hematuria, or renal failure. Urinalysis may demonstrate

a. Casts (hyaline, granular, fatty, waxy, or epithelial cell)
b. Lipiduria—the presence of free lipid or lipid within tubular cells (oval fat bodies)
c. Fatty casts—presence of lipids within casts
d. Free fat globules (suggests a glomerular disorder causing nephrotic syndrome)
e. Urinary cholesterol—on plain microscopy (Maltese cross pattern under polarized light)
f. Triglycerides in urine—Sudan staining

Other blood tests like hemogram, blood sugar, blood urea, serum creatinine, serum albumin and serum cholesterol are done in all cases.

For diagnosing the secondary causes of nephrotic syndrome, the following tests will be useful:

a. Serum glucose or glycosylated Hb (HbA1c)
b. Antinuclear antibodies
c. Hepatitis B and C serologic tests
d. Serum or urine protein electrophoresis
e. Cryoglobulins
f. Rheumatoid factor
g. Serologic test for syphilis
h. HIV antibody test
i. Complement levels (CH50, C3, C4)

Abdominal ultrasonogram may be done if indicated. For adults, renal biopsy is done to identify the type of nephrotic syndrome and it helps in planning the treatment and gives an idea about the prognosis. Please see the chapter on renal diseases in children for indications for biopsy in children.

MANAGEMENT

The general treatment of nephrotic syndrome is by maintaining a fluid balance chart, daily weight recording, fluid and salt restriction to achieve relief of edema and weight loss as desired and restriction of strenuous physical activity. Diuretics should be used carefully because they may cause further loss of water from the intravascular compartment leading to hypotension and renal failure. The diet should provide 35 kcal/kg body weight with normal protein intake and restricted fat intake. The fluid intake is regulated according to the intake output and daily weight chart. The primary disorder causing nephrotic syndrome should be identified and corrected if a secondary cause is present.

The initial treatment is with corticosteroids—prednisolone 1 mg/kg body weight (maximum 80 mg/day) in adults and 2 mg/kg body weight (maximum 60 mg/day) in children. This is given together with antacids or ranitidine (to minimize gastric upset). The treatment is usually continued for 6 weeks and changed to alternate day therapy and gradually tapered. It is not safe to stop long term treatment with steroids suddenly because the patient may develop acute adrenal hormone deficiency if treatment is stopped suddenly. If the patient has no protein loss in urine for 3 consecutive days, it is called remission. Depending on the response, the nephrotic syndrome is included in categories like steroid responsive, steroid dependant, steroid resistant, etc. (Please see the section on nephrotic syndrome in children (Chapter—) for detailed definitions.)

Those who relapse infrequently may be treated with a shorter course of the above dose which is continued till urine protein remains 'NIL' continuously for 3 days. For frequently relapsing nephrotic syndrome, steroid dependant or resistant cases, a renal biopsy is performed and more powerful drugs are tried. The other drugs that can be used in nephrotic syndrome include cyclophosphamide, mycophenolate, cyclosporine or levamisol. Sometimes, proteinuria may not improve with treatment. In such cases, angiotensin converting enzyme inhibitor drugs and NSAIDs are given to reduce protein loss in urine. Hyperlipidemia usually subsides when proteinuria disappears. If hyperlipidemia persists longer, lid lowering drugs like atorvastatin is given. Since these patients are prone to infection, pneumococcal vaccination should be given if possible. Live attenuated vaccines are avoided in patients with suppressed immune response.

COMPLICATIONS

Complications may occur because of the illness or as a result of drugs used for treatment.

Disease Related Complications

a. *Infections:* Bacterial and viral infection occur due to suppressed immune system. Spontaneous bacterial peritonitis, cellulitis or sepsis may occur in nephrotic syndrome commonly.

b. *Thromboembolism:* Clotting of blood in the vein (venous thromboembolism) or artery (arterial thromboembolism) occurs as a complication. This is due to the loss of the normal circulating anticoagulant factors like antithrombin 3 in urine, increased formation of pro-coagulant factors from the liver, sluggish blood flow and increased viscosity (thickening of blood). Those who are prone to develop or those who already have thromboembolic episodes require long-term anticoagulation treatment.

c. *Hypotension:* Occurs because of edema and trapping of the body fluids outside the vascular system. Patient may develop hypotension, shock and acute renal failure. Development of tachycardia and postural hypotension are the early signs which help to diagnose the condition early.

d. *Growth retardation in children:* Due to chronic illness and steroid treatment.

e. Cardiovascular system can be affected by persistent lipid abnormalities.

f. *Anemia and poor nutritional state:* Edematous mucosa in the gastrointestinal system may prevent absorption of nutrients and result in anemia and nutritional deficiency.

g. Hormonal deficiencies occur because of loss in urine.

Complications Related to Treatment

a. *Due to steroid therapy:* Acne, moon facies, osteoporosis, diabetes, obesity, infections, gastric ulcers, growth retardation, cataract, hypertension, psychosis

b. *Cyclophosphamide therapy:* Leucopenia, hemorrhagic cystitis, infertility, hairloss.

c. *Cyclosporin:* Gum hypertrophy, diabetes, hair growth, gum hypertrophy, hypertension and renal failure.

d. *Azathioprine:* Leucopenia, liver enzyme elevation.

Prognosis

The prognosis of children with primary minimal change disease is generally good. In adults also the prognosis is favorable if hematuria, hypertension and renal failure are not present. Some adults with minimal change disease may behave like FSGS. The renal functions in those with FSGS worsen gradually over many years and they may reach 'end stage renal disease' after many years. Some cases of FSGS progress rapidly to renal failure. These cases are called 'malignant FSGS'. Patients with membranous nephropathy may have spontaneous remission (cure), or progress slowly, progress fast or die due to complications. In all cases of nephrotic syndrome associated with the infection, hypertension, renal failure, hematuria or thrombostic tendancy, the long-term prognosis may be poor. In patients with focal segmental glomerulosclerosis, IgA nephropathy, and membranoproliferative glomerulonephritis, the chances of recurrence in transplanted kidney is high.

13

Acute Kidney Injury

R Kasi Visweswaran, Satheesh Balakrishnan

Kidneys are highly susceptible in damage to many factors. Acute kidney injury (AKI) means sudden onset of impairment of renal function (which may occur within a few hours or weeks) leading to retention in blood of substances normally excreted by the kidneys. It is also known as acute renal insufficiency syndrome. Two main types of AKI are recognized. One type is 'community acquired' and the second is 'hospital acquired'. Community acquired occurs due to diseases like gastroenteritis, dehydration, blood loss, snake envenomation, leptospirosis, or use of nephrotoxic toxins or drugs. The common hospital acquired causes are sepsis, hypotension, fluid and electrolyte imbalance, use of many drugs or often a combination of these. If the kidneys alone are affected, the prognosis is good. If multiple organs are affected (multiorgan failure), the prognosis may be poor.

DEFINITION AND CLASSIFICATION

Certain criteria have been laid out for defining AKI. A graded definition of AKI called the risk, injury, failure, loss of function and end stage renal failure, also called 'RIFLE' criteria has been proposed. The 'RIFLE' criteria consists of three graded levels of injury (risk, injury, and failure) based on degree of elevation in serum creatinine or urine output and outcome (Table 13.1).

According to the acute kidney injury network (AKIN) modified criteria, the following points are considered for diagnosis of AKI.

a. An abrupt increase in the serum creatinine concentration of ≥0.3 mg/dl (26.4 µmol/L) from baseline (within 48 hrs),
b. Increase in the serum creatinine concentration by ≥50%.
c. Oliguria <0.5 ml/kg per hour for more than six hours.

Table 13.1: RIFLE Classification			
Stage	Increase in creatinine from baseline	Decrease in GFR %	Urine output
R Risk	1.5 to 2 times	>25%	<0.5 ml/kg/hour for <6 hours
I Injury	2.0–3.0 times	>50%	<0.5 ml/kg/hour for <12 hours
F Failure	>3 times	>75 % S. Cr >4 mg or rise >0.5 mg	<0.3 ml/kg/hour for 24 hours or anuria for 12 hours.
L Loss	Persistent failure needing dialysis		
E End stage	Permanent failure needing dialysis for >3 months		

Another system of classification is based on kidney disease improving global outcome (KDIGO) guidelines. In this, the AKI is divided into 3 stages.

- Stage 1 = Serum creatinine increase 1.5 to 1.9 times baseline or >0.3 mg% in 24 hours or output <0.5 ml/kg/hour for 6 hours
- Stage 2 = 2–2.9 times baseline or <0.5 ml/kg/hour for 12 hours
- Stage 3 = 3 times baseline or creatinine >4 mg% or initiation of dialysis or output <0.3 ml/kg/hour for 12 hours or anuria for 12 hours.

The causes of AKI can be broadly divided into

1. Prerenal causes
2. Intrinsic renal causes and
3. Postrenal causes.

PRERENAL AKI

Prerenal conditions are those conditions where the kidneys do not get adequate quantities of blood (poor renal perfusion). It can be due to the blood volume is low or the blood pressure is low or both. Normal blood pressure is required for glomerular filtration. When low renal perfusion occurs, the filtration is affected and the patient may develop oliguria, electrolyte disturbances and accumulation of waste products in blood. If the defect is identified and corrected immediately, the kidneys will recover, and renal functions will become normal.

Causes of Prerenal Failure

1. Conditions causing low blood volume
   a. Loss of blood—external or internal bleeding
   b. Loss of plasma—burns
   c. Loss of fluids and electrolytes—gastrointestinal fluid losses like gastroenteritis, cholera
   d. 'Third space' fluid loss—intestinal obstruction/paralytic ileus
   e. Loss of water—heat stroke, insufficient water intake
2. Conditions causing low blood pressure (hypotension)
   a. Cardiogenic shock
   b. Septic shock
   c. Severe cardiac failure (pump failure)
   d. Obstruction to flow of blood (massive pulmonary embolism)
   e. Persistence for a long time of all prerenal causes
   f. Drugs causing reduction in glomerular blood flow (cyclosporin, NSAIDs, ACE inhibitors)
3. Hepatorenal syndrome: Cirrhosis of liver with liver failure can cause simultaneous renal failure. This is called hepatorenal syndrome.

When pre-renal remains uncorrected for a long time, the patient may develop kidney damage and the renal tubules undergo necrosis. This stage is called acute tubular necrosis. Usually, it takes a few weeks for the tubules to recover and the patient may need careful treatment including dialysis during this time. Any acute disease involving the tissues in the kidney can cause acute kidney injury.

Intrinsic Renal Causes of AKI

1. Abnormalities of blood vessels in kidney (renal circulation)
   a. Bilateral arterial block
   b. Bilateral venous block
   c. Renal vasculitis (acute inflammation of small blood vessels in the kidney)
   d. Malignant hypertension (sudden and severe increase in blood pressure)
   e. Atheroembolic renal failure (cholesterol embolism, block due to atherosclerosis)

2. Acute diseases of the glomeruli
   a. Acute glomerulonephritis
   b. Rapidly progressive glomerulonephritis
   c. Hemolytic uremic syndrome
3. Abnormalities in renal tubule
   a. Ischemic acute tubular necrosis (if prerenal factors remain uncorrected for a long time, the tubules undergo necrosis because of poor blood supply).
   b. *Toxic tubular necrosis:* It occurs due to nephrotoxic drugs (methotrexate, cisplatin, radiocontrast media), hemoglobin, myoglobin, surgery, trauma, burns or sepsis or other toxic substances.
4. Renal transplant rejection
5. Acute allergic interstitial nephritis (allergy to penicillin, rifampicin, cephalosporin, frusemide, proton pump inhibitors)
6. **Obstetric causes:** Earlier, AKI in early pregnancy was related to septic abortion and use of nephrotoxic abortifacients. In late pregnancy, antepartum or postpartum hemorrhage, abruptio placentae caused AKI. The incidence of AKI in pregnancy has decreased now. Pregnant women with pre-eclampsia and HELLP syndrome can develop AKI.

Postrenal Causes of AKI

Postrenal AKI is seen in hospitalized patients as well as those in the community. It is more common in elderly patients and caused by urinary tract obstruction. Any obstruction to flow of urine can lead to retention of waste products and AKI.

1. Conditions causing urethral obstruction
   a. Stricture of urethra
   b. Posterior urethral valve in children
   c. Urethral stone obstruction
   d. Prostatic hypertrophy in old men
2. Ureteric obstruction to single functioning kidney
3. Bilateral ureteric obstruction
   a. Carcinoma bladder involving vesicoureteric junction
   b. Carcinoma cervix infiltrating to bladder
   c. Bilateral obstructing ureteric calculi
   d. Retroperitoneal fibrosis.

If there is total obstruction, the patient will have anuria (less than 50 ml in one day). If the patient is not passing even a drop of urine, obstruction should be ruled out immediately by physical examination, catheter change and ultrasonography. Block of the urinary catheter is a common situation encountered in the hospital where the patient does not pass even a drop of urine. If the block is in the lower urinary tract, the bladder will be enlarged.

The following persons are at high risk of developing AKI

a. Elderly persons (reduced renal functional capacity)
b. Persons with pre-existing chronic kidney disease
c. Hypertension
d. Diabetes mellitus
e. Hypercholesterolemia
f. Obesity
g. Use of multiple drugs
h. Urinary tract infection
i. Other infections/sepsis

DIAGNOSIS AND MANAGEMENT

Diagnosis can be confirmed by a recent decrease in kidney function—decrease in creatinine clearance (glomerular filtration rate), increase in serum creatinine. Examination of urine for osmolality, sodium, microscopy, serum electrolytes, urea, urine to plasma ratios of urea, creatinine, osmolality help to identify prerenal azotemia from established tubular injury. Imaging studies help diagnose postrenal causes like obstructive uropathy. The patients often go through three phases, the initial oliguric phase, followed by diuretic phase followed by postdiuretic phase. During the oliguric phase, the urine output is low and the renal functions keep on worsening. During the diuretic phase, the renal functions may continue to worsen initially but start improving. During this phase, there may be uncontrollable dieresis due to nonrecovery of tubular function (the function of tubule is to reabsorb 99% of the glomerular filtrate). As the tubule recovers, the patient goes into postdiuretic phase in which renal functions become normal.

In early oliguric phase, when tubular damage has not set in, correction of dehydration and improvement of blood pressure will help the kidneys to recover without going into tubular damage. If there is obstruction, early correction of obstruction using appropriate catheter and drainage of urine will be helpful. The treatment of intrinsic renal failure depends on the cause. Nephrotoxic drugs should be avoided. Fluid balance chart, daily weight recording, salt and fluid restriction, potassium free diet, protein intake limited to 0.8 g/kg, high calorie diet are advised. If hyperkalemia develops, conservative treatment can be tried and if it fails, patient can be taken up for emergency dialysis. Conservative treatment of hyperkalemia is administration of 10 ml calcium gluconate slowly. This helps to stabilize the myocardial membrane and prevent arrhythmia due to hyperkalemia. The next step is to give insulin with glucose. Insulin causes shift of potassium from blood to the intracellular compartment. Glucose is given to prevent hypoglycemic effect of insulin. In those with severe acidosis, sodium bicarbonate injections help to shift the potassium to the intracellular compartment. Salbutamol tablets or nebulisations are also useful in emergencies. Potassium exchang resins and dialysis are the only ways of removing potassium from the body. Hyperkalemia and fluid overload are the important emergency indications for dialysis. There is no specific drug to help kidney function to recover fast. When recovery of function starts, the urine output will start increasing. Usually, there will be doubling in the volume of output every day for a few days before complete recovery of renal functions occur. During the diuretic phase, water restriction is relaxed, patient permitted salt and potassium intake and normal diet. If potassium is not given at this stage, patient may develop hypokalemia. If the oliguric phase is prolonged, and urea, creatinine and potassium are increasing steadily or bicarbonate levels decreasing, dialysis support is necessary. The decision on starting dialysis is taken, based on the general condition of the patient and biochemical values.

Recent developments include some biomarkers which help to suspect kidney injury even before the creatinine shows signs of increasing trend. Thus, they may help in the early diagnosis and treatment of AKI. These molecules are urine interlukin 18 (IL-18), urine neutrophil gelatinase-associated lipocalin (NGAL), plasma NGAL, cystatin C, or kidney injury molecule-1 (KIM-1).

14

Chronic Kidney Disease

Reena Thomas, R Kasi Visweswaran

Chronic kidney disease (CKD) is a very common problem seen worldwide. The definition of CKD is as follows. CKD is defined as the presence of kidney damage or an estimated or measured glomerular filtration rate (GFR) of less than 60 ml/min/1.73 m^2 for a period greater than 3 months. Kidney disease means abnormalities of urine sediment, abnormal results of imaging tests, or if the patient has had a kidney biopsy with documented abnormalities. CKD can be diagnosed even though the GFR is over 60 ml/min/1.73 m^2. CKD and renal failure are not the same.

The markers of kidney damage are:

1. Albuminuria > 30 mg/day
2. Abnormalities in urine microscopy
3. Abnormalities in renal function tests
4. Abnormalities in renal imaging
5. Abnormalities in renal pathology
6. After renal transplantation.

A person with any of the above is considered to have CKD even if the GFR is normal if the problem is present for more than 3 months. Patients GFR <60 ml/min are considered as CKD stage 3, even if they have none of the above markers of renal damage.

ETIOLOGY OF CKD

Diabetes is the leading cause of CKD. Other common causes are chronic glomerulonephritis, chronic interstitial nephritis and hypertension. These constitute about 75% of the causes of CKD (Fig. 14.1).

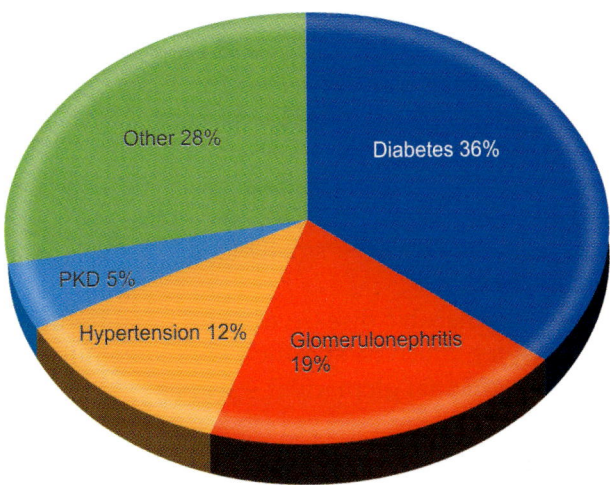

Fig. 14.1: Common causes of CKD

Kidney diseases causing CKD can be classified as

1. *Congenital causes of abnormal kidneys (renal anomalies)*
   a. Obstructive uropathy (obstruction to the urinary tract)
   b. Posterior urethral valve (valve like tissue in the posterior part of urethra which will obstruct free flow of urine)
   c. Pelviureteric junction obstruction (narrowing at the junction of renal pelvis and ureter causing block and enlargement and bulging of pelvis, calyces and kidney)
   d. Renal aplasia or hypoplasia (nondevelopment or poor development of the kidney. The kidney may be absent or small and poorly or not functioning)
   e. Reflux neuropathy (damage to kidney due to back flow of urine from bladder during urination)
   f. Polycystic kidney disease (congenital and inherited diseases where the kidneys contain many cysts. The cysts grow as the child grows and may cause symptoms only by 30–40 years of age. Some cysts may cause renal failure earlier).

2. *Vascular diseases*
   a. Bilateral renal artery stenosis (renal arteries on both sides are narrowed resulting in poor blood supply to kidney. The kidneys secrete renin when blood supply is decreased and fail when blood supply is inadequate).

   b. Ischemic nephropathy (there is ischemia to both kidneys often due to atherosclerosis of aorta and renal arteries)

   c. Hemolytic uremic syndrome (condition associated with acute kidney injury which may not recover, it is due to damage to glomerulus)

   d. Vasculitis (inflammatory disease involving all types of blood vessels. It may be large vessel like aorta and its branches, medium-sized vessels or small blood vessels)

3. *Glomerular diseases*

   a. Primary glomerular disease (diseases mainly affecting the glomeruli for which no specific cause is identified)

     i. Focal segmental glomerular sclerosis

     ii. IgA nephropathy

     iii. Membranoproliferative glomerular nephritis

     iv. Membranous nephropathy

   b. Secondary glomerular disease

     i. Diabetes mellitus

     ii. Hypertension

     iii. Collagen group of diseases

4. *Tubulointerstitial disease*

   a. Drugs

   b. Toxins

   c. Chronic pyelonephritis

   d. Reflux neuropathy.

   e. Renal tumors (most renal tumors arise from the tubule or epithelial cell)

5. *Obstructive uropathy*

   a. Bilateral renal calculi

   b. Prostatic enlargement.

It is important to diagnose CKD early and prevent the progression. People who have high-risk for developing CKD, should be regularly screened and periodically followed up. The following persons at high-risk and should be screened and if they have evidence of CKD, they should be advised annual follow-up.

- Family history of CKD/renal failure
- Family history of hypertension
- Family history of diabetes mellitus
- Family history of inherited kidney disease
- Past history of acute kidney injury

- Patients with cardiovascular disease
- Patients with kidney stones or an enlarged prostate.
- Patients with multi-systemic disease like lupus erythematosus.
- Patients with urinary abnormalities (hematuria, proteinuria or pyuria).

STAGING OF RENAL FAILURE

Assessment of renal function is an important step in the staging of CKD. Serum creatinine and urea are the usual laboratory tests to diagnose renal failure. Blood urea level may change with change in diet, dehydration and other factors. Creatinine level is usually steady. Creatinine level does not change very much in the early stages of renal failure. The serum creatinine will increase from 1 mg% to 2 mg% only when the kidney function reduces from 100% to 50%. When the creatinine doubles, the GFR reduces by 50%. Hence, serum creatinine cannot be used to reliably assess GFR in early stages of renal failure. GFR is a more reliable way to assess the working of the kidneys. GFR is a measure of how much volume of fluid is filtered by the kidney every minute. It is expressed as ml/min. A healthy pair of kidneys should be able to filter about 90–120 ml/min. Depending on the level of GFR, CKD is staged. The alphabet G is used for staging GFR, A for albuminuria and D for dialysis (Table 14.1).

Table 14.1: Criteria for staging CKD		
Stage	*GFR-ml/ min/1.73 m²*	*Remarks*
G 1	≥90	Normal kidney function—only markers present*
G 2	60–89	Normal kidney function—only markers present*
G 3a	45–59	CKD 3a even if markers of kidney damage are absent
G 3b	30–44	CKD 3b even if markers of kidney damage are absent
G 4	15–29	CKD 4 even if markers of kidney damage are absent
G 5	<15	CKD 5 even if markers of kidney damage are absent. If on dialysis, add D.

*Depending on the severity of albuminuria, use prefix A

A1 = Albuminuria <30 mg/day (normal range of urinary albumin excretion)

A2 = Albuminuria = 30–299 mg/day moderate increase but not detected by simple lab tests

A3 = Albuminuria >300 mg/day detected by simple lab tests.

ESTIMATION OF GFR

A bedside estimation of GFR can be made with the Cockcroft-Gault equation and the Schwartz formula in children. There are other equations like the Modification of Diet in Renal Disease (MDRD) formula which is a computer-based one. Since the values of GFR may fluctuate, the diagnosis of CKD may be confirmed only if repeated GFR tests show low levels consistently over three months.

Cockcroft-Gault formula:

$$\text{Creatinine clearance} = \frac{(140 - \text{age in years}) \times (\text{body weight in kg})}{72 \times \text{serum creatinine in mg/dl}}$$

• To determine the GFR in a woman, multiply the result by 0.85.

CLINICAL MANIFESTATIONS

Any system of the body can be affected when kidneys fail. Since the disease usually progresses slowly, the body adapts easily to the changes in the internal environment and remains without symptoms till the patients are in advanced renal failure. This is the importance of screening and follow-up patients at risk for renal failure or from the time of diagnosis.

Hypertension is the most common manifestation and is due to sodium and water retention or due to activation of the renin angiotensin system. Most patients develop edema and oliguria towards the later stages.

Cutaneous manifestations include pallor, swallow complexion, dry skin with itching and pigmentation. Intense pruritis (itching) occurs in severe renal failure with excoriation of skin due to scratching. Kryle's disease or prurigo nodularis is presence of hyperkeratotic papules in the skin associated with intense itching and scratching. Uremic frost is a condition where the urea excreted through the sweat precipitates on the skin surface.

Nail changes include pitting, half and half nails with proximal white and distal pink color.

Eye changes include red eye (due to calcium deposition, irritation and bleeding in conjunctiva), band keratopathy (due to calcium deposition in the cornea as a band in the exposed area of the cornea).

Gastrointestinal manifestations are nausea, vomiting, loss of appetite, macroglossia and uremic fetor (smell of urine in breath). The patient may develop GI ulcers and metallic taste in the mouth. **Cardiovascular** manifestations include pericarditis, pericardial effusion or tamponade. In pericardial tamponade, fluid or blood collects in the pericardial cavity and compress the heart. Thus the cardiac function is affected. This occurs only in patients with advanced renal failure. There is a high incidence of cardiovasccular disease and is mainly due to lipid abnormalities atherosclerosis and vascular calcification. When the calcium and phosphorus are higher, calcification may occur in tissues. If the Ca × P product is more than 70, calcification can occur in other tissues.

Example: Serum Ca = 9.5 mg% and phosphorus = 4 mg%.

Ca × P (product) = 9.5 × 4 = 38.

Serum Ca = 9.0 mg% and phosphorus = 8.0 mg%

Ca × P (product) = 9.5 × 8 = 76.

Since the product is > 70, chances of calcification are high.

Neuropsychiatric manifestations include paresthesia, peripheral neuropathy, flapping tremor, restless legs syndrome, uremic encephalopathy with coma and seizures. Sleep problems due to muscle cramps or restless legs may be present. The patient may develop personality changes and depression.

Respiratory symptoms are due to acidosis and pulmonary edema. In acidosis, the patient will have deep and fast breathing. This type of breathing is called Kussmaul's breathing. When there is pulmonary edema, the patient will have dyspnea and orthopnea. Pulmonary edema may occur due to uncontrolled hypertension and volume overload.

Hematological changes include anemia due to iron deficiency or decreased erythropoietin production in the kidney. The life span of the RBCs is reduced and the bone marrow is suppressed due to uremic toxins. Nutritional factors also play a part in causing anemia due to dietary restriction and decreased appetite of the patient. Anemia due to iron deficiency is commonly associated with normocytic, normochromic anemia due to EPO deficiency. Bleeding tendency occurs due to platelet dysfunction.

Immunity is also impaired with higher susceptibility to infections.

Thus, the patient may present to any department with appropriate symptom. Unless suspected, early diagnosis may be difficult. Patient may seek treatment from gynecologist for sterility or irregular periods, urologist for male sterility, impotence or oligozoospermia, orthopedic surgeon for vague bone pains, neurologist for neuropsychiatric manifestations, hematologist for anemia or bleeding tendency, cardiologist for pericarditis, chest pain or related symptoms, gastroenterologist for upper abdominal symptoms or pulmonologist with dyspnea.

MANAGEMENT

The management should be started early so that worsening of renal failure can be delayed. The first step is to identify and correct the reversible factors. This will help in preventing or slowing the progression of renal disease.

1. **Diet:** The diet is very important and should contain sufficient calories and proteins. A minimum of 35–40 kcal/kg body weight and 0.6–0.8 g protein/kg are essential. At least 50% of prescribed protein should be of high biological value and should be distributed in all the meals for better utilisation. If protein intake is below than this, it may result in negative nitrogen balance and is harmful for the patient. Since most of our patients are already on low protein diet, protein restriction as suggested for patients in other countries is not necessary. Our diet together with egg white and fish may be advised. Red meat should be avoided. Controlling dietary phosphorus is important at all stages of kidney disease. In many cases reducing protein intake will also reduce phosphorus intake. Heavy nonvegetarian diet is a source of acid ions, proteins and phosphates. In advanced renal failure the protein intake should not exceed 0.8 g/kg/day. More important is salt and fluid restriction which will prevent edema formation. Nitrogen free analogues (ketoanalogues) of essential amino acids help to utilise the nitrogen in the body for producing the essential amino acids. These are not very palatable and also expensive but may be useful in delaying the dialysis. In advanced renal failure, potassium restriction is also necessary since the patients may develop hyperkalemia which is an emergency. Potassium content in food items is shown in Table 14.2.

Table 14.2: Potassium content in various food items	
Foods low in potassium: – (Group 1)	– Rice, semolina (rawa) vegetables such as cucumber, ridge gourd, snake gourd, tinda, broad beans, beetroot, fenugreek leaves (methi), green mango, pink radish, bottle gourd – Fruit such as apple (1/4), pineapple (1/4), guava, papaya, pear. – Chicken and meat-boiled in excess water twice and drained. – Egg white. – Tea.
Foods moderate in potassium: – (Group 2)	– Rice flakes, corn flakes, bambino vermicelli – Vegetables such as carrot, cauliflower, lady finger, tomatoes, bitter gourd, onions, cabbage, white radish, pumpkin, brinjal, French beans. – Curd – Watermelon, grapes.
Foods high in potassium: – (Group 3)	– Barley, ragi, wheat flour. – All pulses – All leafy vegetables such as amaranth, coriander leaves, drumstick leaves, spinach; potato, colocasia, sweet potato, yam, drumstick, green papaya, sword beans. – Milk, fish especially sardines – Nuts such as cashew nuts, almonds, etc; oilseeds such as peanuts. – Condiments and spices, jaggery. – Fruits such as sweet lime, mango, banana, chickoo, apricots, dates, figs, melons, oranges, pears – Brown sugar, coffee, cocoa powder, chocolate.

2. **Blood pressure control:** The blood pressure must be maintained below 140/90 mmHg. The drugs used are usually angiotensin converting enzyme inhibitors (ACEi), angiotensin receptor blockers (ARBs), direct renin inhibitors (DRIs), calcium channel blockers (CCBs), alpha blockers, beta blockers or diuretics are used for control of hypertension. The dose is adjusted to maintain the blood pressure below 140/90. The selection of the drug and the dose will vary from patient to patient.

3. **Control of hyperphosphatemia, hypocalcemia and high parathyroid hormone:** And low active vitamin D—abnormalities of calcium, phosphorus, parathyroid hormone (PTH), or vitamin D metabolism occur in CKD. When kidney function decreases, phosphorous excretion by the kidney is diminished and active vitamin D synthesis are diminished. This results in hypocalcemia and hyperparathyroidism. Limiting phosphorus intake or preventing its absorption form the GIT helps to break the above chain of events. Milk and meat are sources of high phosphate and hence avoided. Drugs like calcium acetate, calcium carbonate, sevelemer, lanthanum carbonate are given with food so that they bind with the phosphorus and prevent the absorption. Depending on the calcium level, active vitamin D as calcitriol (1, 25-dihydroxy cholecalciferol) can be used.

4. **Control of hyperuricemia:** Since uric acid cannot be excreted by the diseased kidney, it will accumulate. Uric acid is toxic to many tissues in the body. Hence drugs to reduce uric acid like allopurinol of febuxostat are given. Alkalies help to excrete more of the end products. So alkalies are also given with uric acid lowering drugs.

5. **Control acidosis and prevent bone resorption:** Chronic acidosis will result in using up the body buffers. Bicarbonate in blood is an important immediate buffering system. Later, the bone buffer is used up resulting in weakness of bones and a condition called uremic renal osteodystrophy. To prevent and treat chronic acidosis, bicarbonate supplements are used. Sodium bicarbonate tablets are used. When given orally, they cause bloated feeling in the abdomen due to release of carbon dioxide. Shohl's solution is a combination of sodium citrate and citric acid. 1 ml of solution will provide 1 mmol of bicarbonate. When anyone is using Shohl's solution, aluminium utensils should not be used for cooking.

6. **Other important aspects in treatment of advanced renal failure are:**
   a. Correction of iron, vitamin B and folic acid deficiency
   b. Replacement of erythropoietin by recombinant human erythropoietin
   c. Control of primary disease
   d. Correct lipid abnormalities

e. Appropriate dosage modification of drugs
f. Protect with hepatitis B vaccination
g. Other vaccinations may be needed for those planning to undergo renal transplantation.

When the renal function is below 20%, the patient must be prepared for renal replacement therapy. The options are long-term hemodialysis, continuous ambulatory peritoneal dialysis or renal transplantation. For long-term hemodialysis, a vascular access should be created early and given time (about 2 months) to mature. If preparations are made early, further treatment can be carried out smoothly.

15

Stone Disease

R Kasi Visweswaran

Stones in the urinary tract have been known from ancient times. Stones have been found in Egyptian mummies and operation for stone has been described in ancient India many centuries before modern medicine came into existence. The stones consist of a nucleus of organic matter or foreign substance around which salt accumulates and the whole structure is held together by a matrix. Kidney stones are endemic in some parts of the world. The kidney stone belt region of world is located in countries of Middle East, North Africa, and Mediterranean region, parts of Pakistan and North Eastern states of India. The stone belt regions are those where the climate is hot and the water contains more calcium. Many factors are responsible for the high incidence of stone disease in these areas. It is more common in young males. Seasonal, socioeconomic, occupational, hereditary and geographical factors play an important role in formation of stones. Individuals with family history of stone disease have three times high-risk of developing kidney stones compared to those without a family history for the disease. Diet containing high calcium, red meat, oxalate and reduce fluid intake, favour stone formation. Kidney stones are formed by end products of metabolism of uric acid, phosphates and oxalates which precipitate in the urine and take shape of stone. Stone disease is a common disease worldwide.

There are two types of stones

1. Primary stones which include stones of calcium, oxalate, uric acid, cystine and xanthine.

2. Secondary stones are formed by urea splitting organisms such as Proteus, Pseudomonas or Klebsiella species. They

are tripple phosphate stones known as struvite stones and are composed of calcium, magnesium and ammonium phosphates.

Stones can vary between the size of a few millimeters to the size of a tennis ball or bigger. Most of the smaller stones may be passed in the urine. Only some stones can be dissolved by medications. A patient with a stone episode has chances of recurrence within the first five years. Urine contains factors which inhibit and favor stone formation. The inhibiting factors are more than stone forming factors. If the balance is tilted in favor of stone formation, stone diseases may develop.

FACTORS INHIBITING STONE FORMATION

1. Dilute urine
2. Constant flow of urine
3. Presence of citrate in urine
4. Presence of magnesium, zinc, pyrophosphates in urine.

FACTORS FAVORING STONE FORMATION COULD BE METABOLIC TO OTHER FACTORS

1. Hyperoxaluria
2. Hypercalciuria
3. Hyperuricosuria
4. Hyperparathyroidism
5. Cystinuria
6. Decrease in inhibitors (as above)
7. Chronic urinary tract infection
8. Congenital anomalies which cause obstruction/stasis.
9. Concentrated urine
10. Neurogenic bladder
11. Familial factors
12. Residence in 'stone belt' areas.

Stone may form in any part of the urinary system. Often they are formed in the kidney and pass down to ureter, bladder or urethra. Usually a stone is formed over a nucleus (nidus). This can be a foreign body, catheter, damaged mucosa. Crystals accumulate over the nidus if the urine is concentrated and saturated with the substance. Thus, the nidus grows into a stone. For secondary calculi, infection is the main cause.

The three main types of stones commonly encountered are:

1. **Oxalate stone (Fig. 15.1):** This is the commonest type and contains calcium salts. Therefore, they can be seen in the X-ray (radiopaque). It may produce pain (colic) and hematuria. When passed or removed, it is usually brownish black in color and has an irregular surface with sharp projections. These types of stones may occur as pure stones or combined with phosphate or uric acid.

2. **Phosphate stone:** Many types of phosphate stones are present. Calcium phosphate stones are formed in alkaline urine. They occur in patients who have infections due to urea splitting organisms which causes alkaline urine. These stones are large and develop the shape of the renal collecting system within which they form. They form staghorn calculi (Fig. 15.2) of triple phosphate (calcium, magnesium and ammonium). Since their surface is smooth, even large staghorn calculi may remain asymptomatic. Because of the presence of some calcium, they may be faintly radiopaque.

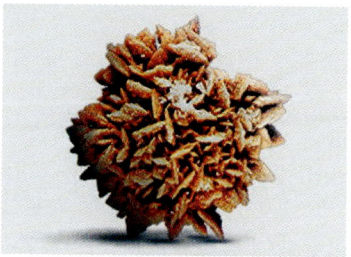

Fig. 15.1: Oxalate stone

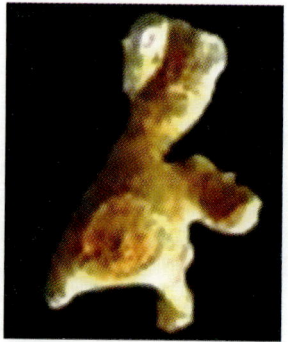

Fig. 15.2: Staghorn calculus—note the shape

3. **Uric acid/urate stone:** Pure uric acid stones occur as a result of abnormalities in uric acid metabolism. The stones form when the urinary excretion of uric acid is high and the urine is acidic. Uric acid stones occur in association with other stones. These are the only types of stones that can be dissolved by prolonged treatment. Most other types of stones cannot be dissolved by medical treatment. The diet preferred in uric acid stone is alkaline diet and low purine (red meat). Fluid intake is increased. Oral alkalie supplements and allopurinol or febuxostat is given for many months.

Cystine stones are rare and occur in cystinuria. Patients take up the diuretic triamterene may develop stone diseases following its long-term use.

The clinical features of stone depend on the position, size, and whether it produces bleeding, colic, obstruction or infection. Asymptomatic small stones in the renal parenchyma do not require aggressive investigations or treatment. Such patients may be periodically followed up. Symptoms may occur due to destruction of renal parenchyma and the patient may have pain, pyuria or hematuria. The renal area may be tender to gentle percussion over the area.

Patients with stones in the ureter usually have colicky pain or 'ureteric colic'. It is a sharp shooting pain from the loin to groin and is associated with vomiting, sweating and sometimes microscopic or macroscopic hematuria. The patient is not comfortable in any position. Sometimes patients experience constant dull pain in the loin only. There may be tenderness on palpation or gentle percussion. Even large bladder stone may remain with no symptom. Some may experience suprapubic pain, frequent urge to pass urine, symptoms due to infections or hematuria towards the end of micturition.

Examination of urine pH helps to suspect some types of stones. Oxalate and uric acid crystals are formed in acid urine. Triple phosphate stones form in alkaline urine and calcium phosphate stones form in neutral urine. If the urine is concentrated, the chances of stone formation and stone growth are more. If urine specific gravity is constantly >1020, there is more chance for stone formation, whereas if it is <1010, chances of stone formation or growth of stone is less.

When we study the urine deposit under the microscope, we can identify the various crystals in the urine. Metabolic stone work up is done to study blood and urine chemistry. Estimation of blood and 24-hr urine levels for calcium, phosphorous, oxalate, uric acid, magnesium, citrate, urea and creatinine are helpful in arriving at a diagnosis, planning diet and treatment for these patients.

Urine culture, abdominal ultrasonography, plain X-ray of abdomen, intravenous urogram, cystography and CT urography are performed as needed.

From the point of view of treatment, it is useful to classify the stones into the following categories.

'Surgically' Active Stone

A surgically active stone is the one which produces pain, obstruction, persistence of infection or bleeding. Such stones have to be managed by any intervention.

'Radiologically' Active Stone

If there is evidence of increase in size, number or repeated passage of stones or gravel, it is called radiologically active.

'Metabolically' Active Stone

A metabolically active stone is one which is associated with significant biochemical abnormally in blood or urine. A metabolically active stone will require modification of diet and use of drugs to prevent further increase in size or number. Rarely some stones like uric acid stones can be dissolved with the use of medicines for many months.

'Indeterminate Metabolic Activity'

A stone which is recently diagnosed and is not surgically active should be considered in this category. Only after observing such stone for 1 year, we will be able to decide if it is radiologically or metabolically active.

Metabolically Inactive Stone

This term is used for a stone which has remained silent, has not increased in size or number and has caused no symptoms for more than 1 year.

TREATMENT

General Treatment

The commonest disabling symptom due to stone is pain due to ureteric colic. It is a pain of undescribable severity and the patients need a combination of antispasmodics and NSAIDs. If there is obstruction, it has to be relieved at the earliest. In severe cases, narcotic analgesics may be given. However, we must be careful about using such drugs because of addiction. Some patients who have received one dose of pethidine have come back malingering severe pain!! Good fluid intake to stimulate good urine flow can also help to improve the pain. The flow of urine not only helps to expel the stone but may also protect the mucosa from contact with the rough edges of the stone.

Special diets are given if the types of stones are known. Increasing fluid intake and maintaining urine specific gravity below 1010 is useful. Since the patients cannot measure specific gravity on their own, the practical advise is to give adequate fluids so that urine ouput is over 3000 ml in 24 hours.

For uric acid stones associated with high serum uric acid level, use of Allopurinol 200–300 mg/day combined with alkalinisation of urine continuously for 1–2 yrs is advised. This helps to dissolve uric acid stones. In the case of cystinuria with cystine stones, D-penicillamine in dose of 750–1250 mg/day is used to dissolve the cystine stones.

Methods of removal of stone from the body are divided into:

a. Nonsurgical
b. Surgical

Nonsurgical Method

In earlier days, open surgical methods were only available. Now nonsurgical methods are available. They are as follows.

Extracorporeal Shock Wave Lithotripsy (ESWL)

It is ideal for stones in kidney and upper urinary tract. The shock waves produced outside the body are directed to focus on the stone inside the body and the stones are broken to small fragments. The powdered stone and small fragments are eliminated through the urinary tract.

Percutaneous Nephrolithotomy (PCNL)

The dilated collecting system of the kidney is reached through a needle in the renal angle. After passing a guidewire, the track is dilated to enable the passage of the nephroscope. The surgeon is able to visualize the stone and remove it through the scope.

Ureterorenoscopy (URS)

The patient first undergoes cystoscopy. Through the cystoscope the URS is introduced into the ureter and advanced till the stone is reached. Thereafter it can be powdered by using ultrasound wave, electrohydraulic shock waves or laser beams. If the stone is impacted near the lower end of ureter, a basket-like device (Dormia basket) is used to pull it out through the urinary passage.

Cystolithotripsy

A stone in the bladder can be visualized through the cystoscope, broken or crushed using lithotripter (crushing forceps).

Surgical Methods

Pyelolithotomy

The stone in the renal pelvis is removed surgically by opening the renal pelvis. This can be done by open or laparoscopic surgery.

Nephrolithotomy

If the stone is in the renal calyx, the renal cortex overlying the calyx is opened and the stone removed through the opening.

Ureterolithotomy

It refers to open removal of stone in ureter directly through a small incision in the ureter.

Cystolithotomy

It is the surgical procedure where the urinary bladder is cut open to remove the stone.

Since less invasive nonsurgical methods are available now, surgical methods are not used commonly.

16

Asymptomatic Urinary Abnormalities (AUA)

R Kasi Visweswaran

The person may be totally asymptomatic but on routine checkup, insurance, employment or basic investigations for other diseases, the urine examination may show some abnormality. Some of these may not be significant but sometimes it may indicate significant illness or may be an early sign of a serious disorder. Therefore anyone having significant abnormalities in urine examinations must be investigated appropriately and also followed up. Presence of protein, blood or RBG, WBCs or pus cells, crystals, casts, bacteria in the urine in a person who is totally asymptomatic is included as AUA. If any urinary abnormality persists for over 3 months, the patient is considered to have chronic kidney disease as per the current definition irrespective of whether the renal function is normal or abnormal.

MICROSCOPIC HEMATURIA

It is the presence of >5 RBCs in a high power field under the microscope in a properly collected and processed sample of urine. Glomerular diseases like IqA nephropathy, Alport's syndrome, thin basement membrane disease and subclinical acute nephritis are the common conditions associated with RBG in urine microscopy. Other causes of blood in urine like acute nephritis, renal tumors, infections or injuries often have some symptoms.

PROTEINURIA

Routine examination of urine may show presence of protein. Normal urine contains a small quantity of protein which includes Tamm-Horsfall mucoprotein secreted by tubular cells, immunoglobulin fragments and less than 30 mg albumin in 24 hrs.

The daily urine protein excretion is <150 mg. If it is more than >500 mg, it can be detected easily by simple laboratory tests. Asymptomatic proteinuria may be due to orthostatic proteinuria. In orthostatic proteinuria, there is no proteinuria when the person is lying down. The urine formed when the person is ambulant and active will have proteinuria. Various glomerular diseases are associated with proteinuria. In glomerular involvement, the proteinuria is more severe and the 24-hr urine may show >1.5 g/day. In nephrotic syndrome, 24-hr urine protein is 3.5 g/day. In tubular diseases and infection, the severity of proteinuria is lesser (<1.5 g/day).

Asymptomatic Bacteriuria

This means the presence of bacteria in the urine in a person who has no symptoms of urinary tract infection. The urine culture grows >10^5 colony forming units/ml of urine. Except in the case of asymptomatic bacteriuria in pregnancy, elderly diabetes or children with vesicoureteric reflux (passage of urine from bladder, back to the ureter during micturition), no active treatment is required. Follow up is essential for all patients.

Asymptomatic Pyuria

May occur in partially treated urinary tract infections, prostatitis, genitourinary tuberculosis, early stages of tumors, and some drugs. Further tests are required to identify the cause of pyuria. Tuberculosis is associated with "Acid sterile pyunia". In this condition the urine may be acidic in reaction, with pyuria but the routine urine culture will be always sterile.

Presence of various crystals may signify some biochemical abnormalities and such patients must be investigated appropriately. Presence of oxalate crystals, cystine crystals and uric acid crystal may signify abnormalities in the metabolism and elimination of these substances.

17

Cysts in the Kidney

Reena Thomas, R Kasi Visweswaran

Many types of cysts are seen in the kidneys. Most of them may be detected on examination of the abdomen by ultrasonography or scanning. Cysts are fluid-filled swellings present in any part of the body. When they are present in the kidneys, they are called renal cysts. They may vary in size from very small microscopic cyst to very large ones. The number can vary from one to many thousands. The cyst can be simple or complex. A complex cyst may be infected, have bleeding, calcification or rarely be a tumor or cancer. Simple cysts may be single or multiple. In some diseases the cysts may be so large and numerous and the kidneys may be very large.

CLASSIFICATION OF RENAL CYSTS

A. Genetic
B. Nongenetic

The commonest genetic cysts inherited from parent to offspring in autosomal dominant polycystic kidney disease (ADPKD). It is a very common disease which runs in families and often causes renal failure after middle age. von Hippel-Lindau (vHL) disease, tuberous sclerosis (TSC)—other causes of cysts in the kidney which are inherited as autosomal dominant. Autosomal recessive polycystic kidney disease (ARPKD) is not as common as ADPKD and is inherited as an autosomal recessive pattern of inheritance. Other conditions like juvenile nephronophthisis and orofaciodigital syndrome type 1 are also inherited in an autosomal recessive pattern.

Nongenetic renal cysts may be developmental anomalies like medullary sponge kidney or acquired conditions like simple cysts,

cysts that develop following renal failure, dialysis or in chronic hypokalemia.

Cysts seen in neonatal period and infancy are ARPKD, TSC, and rarely ADPKD. The renal cysts in adolescent age group are juvenile nephronophthisis, medullary cystic disease, ARPKD and ADPKD. In adults, ADPKD, MSK, simple cysts, acquired cystic disease of kidney, VHL occur. If the renal cysts are associated with other congenital abnormalities, VHL, TSC should be considered.

ADPKD

ADPKD is a progressive disorder affecting kidneys and other systems characterized by the formation and gradual enlargement of cysts in the kidney. Other organs like liver, pancreas, spleen, lung or epididymis may be affected. It is common and may occur in approximately 1 in 1000 live births. The cysts may be microscopic at birth. As the child grows, the cysts also grow. The disease is characterised by fluid filled cysts of varying sizes arising from the tubules and collecting ducts of both kidneys. The number of cysts may be even thousands. In ultrasonography, presence of at least 6 cysts on each side is necessary for the diagnosis. Manifestations outside the urinary system are liver, lung or pancreatic cysts, hypertension, heart valve defects, aneurysms of the arteries in the brain. Sometimes, these aneurism bursts leading in intracerebral hemorrhage and the diagnosis of ADPKD may be made only then.

Mutation of two genes is responsible for ADPKD. They are PKD 1 gene in chromosome 16 and PKD2 gene in chromosome 4. These genes control proteins known as polycystin 1 and 2 which control the cell functions (cell to cell and cell to matrix interactions, activity of the cilia in cells). Cyst formation involves increased cell proliferation, fluid accumulation and basement membrane remodeling.

Study of the kidney by pathological examination shows both kidneys to be enormously enlarged with numerous cysts throughout the cortex and medulla (Fig. 17.1). There will be distortion of the pelvicalyceal system. Cysts can vary from very small to several centimeters. The kidney may weigh several kilograms. The cysts are lined by a simple cuboidal epithelium and are filled with fluid.

Young patients may be asymptomatic but on examination, the kidneys may be enlarged and palpable. Such patients must be

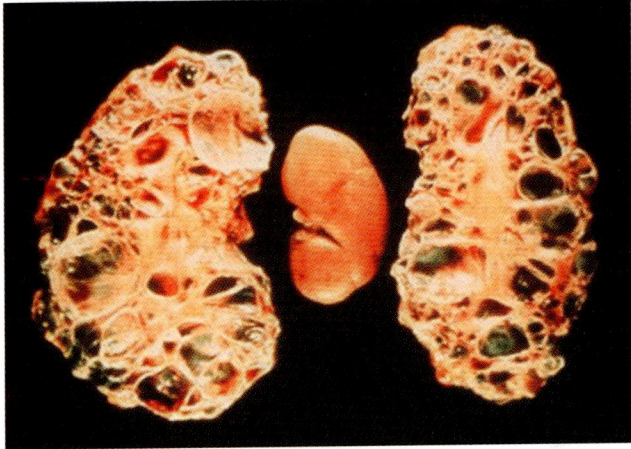

Fig. 17.1: ADPKD—kidneys shown against normal kidney in the middle (autopsy specimens). Note the enlarged kidneys and hundreds of cysts

checked periodically for development of hypertension or renal failure even though there is no symptom. The patient usually presents in the 3rd or 4th decade of life or may be detected earlier as a part of family screening. Family screening is done when another member of the family has ADPKD. Kidney function may worsen progressively due to distortion, compression or other changes in the kidney. Some patients are diagnosed when they present with hypertension at a young age.

The usual symptoms are:

1. *Pain:* The pain is dull, constant and dragging loin pain. If there is infection, bleeding or sudden increase in the size of the cyst, sharp loin pain may occur. Sometimes the pain may be similar to pain due to stone.

2. *Hematuria:* Bleeding in the kidney is usually gross and recurrent and sometimes associated with loin pain. Normally, hematuria subsides by itself with rest.

3. *Bleeding into the cyst:* Blood vessels may rupture and bleed into the cyst causing sudden worsening of pain on the affected side.

4. *Urinary tract infection:* In patients with ADPKD there may be some pus cells in the urine even if there is no infection of urinary tract. This is called sterile pyunia. Urinary tract infection is common in ADPKD. Females are more affected.

The organisms are mainly *E. coli,* Klebsiella, or Proteus species. These infections are treated just like urinary tract infection in adults.

5. *Cyst infection:* Cysts get infected by spread through the blood stream. It manifests as fever and loin pain. The diagnosis is confirmed by ultrasound or CT scans. Cyst aspiration for culture helps to confirm the diagnosis and plan the treatment. Those with cyst infection may need antibiotics which are capable of concentrating in the cyst. The antibiotic treatment should be continued for a few weeks for cure of infection.

6. *Stone disease:* The formation of stones due to calcium and uric acid are very common in patients with ADPKD. The diagnosis and treatment are similar to other patients with stone diseases. Since the kidneys are filled with cysts, surgical and nonsurgical procedures may be technically difficult.

7. Hypertension is very common. It may be the first sign to suspect ADPKD. If a young person presents with hypertension or has secondary hypertension due to renal disease, family history, physical examination and investigations are performed to confirm or exclude the diagnosis of ADPKD.

8. *Renal failure:* Many patients with ADPKD develop pro-gressive renal failure after the age of 50 years. In ADPKD 1 (affected genes in chromosome 16), the illness is more severe. Such patients may develop renal failure earlier. Those with ADPKD 2 (affected gene in chromosome 4), the severity is less and patients remain relatively well in spite of thousands of cysts in each kidney.

9. *Extrarenal manifestations:* In addition to renal manifesta-tions above, the following extrarenal manifestations may occur.

   a. Polycystic liver disease
   b. Intracranial aneurisms (if there is a family member with intracranial aneurism, the chances of aneurisms in the others is high).
   c. Dissection of aorta or major blood vessels
   d. Coronary artery aneurism
   e. Prolapse of cardiac valves
   f. Cysts in other organs: Pancreas, spleen, ovary, seminal vesicle and testes.

Diagnosis

The diagnosis is easy in those who have a sibling or parent with confirmed ADPKD and have both kidneys enlarged and palpable or when renal cysts are associated with hepatic cysts or cerebral aneurism. The diagnosis of ADPKD can be confirmed in persons with family history even if 2 cysts are seen in each kidney by ultrasonography. The number of visible cysts will increase as the age advances. In those with no family history, at least 6 cysts should be present for confirming a diagnosis.

Treatment

There is no specific treatment for the condition. Proper follow up, control of hypertension prevention and treatment of complications are the important goals of therapy. Genetic counseling and screening of all family members will help in early diagnosis. Such persons can be monitored with periodic screening for blood pressure, renal functions and occurrence of complications. Treatment for renal failure can be instituted early because, the diagnosis can be made early by family screening. In patients who develop advanced renal failure, renal replacement therapy will be necessary.

ACQUIRED CYSTIC DISEASE

Patients who remain on dialysis for a long time may develop multiple cysts in the kidney. It is usually distinguished from ADPKD, since there will be family history and the kidneys are small or normal in size with a smooth contour. By contrast, kidneys in ADPKD are markedly enlarged, contain many cysts and may have other cyst in other organs.

AUTOSOMAL RECESSIVE POLYCYSTIC KIDNEY DISEASE (ARPKD)

ARPKD is seen in older children or young adults. It is associated with bulging of collecting duct (ectasia) with cystic changes, nephrolithiasis (stones in kidney), hypertension and sometimes renal failure. These patients have symptoms and signs of hepatic fibrosis and portal hypertension or ascending cholangitis. In the neonatal period, there may be enlarged echogenic kidneys and pulmonary hypoplasia. The occurrence of the disease is controlled by the gene PKHD1 (polycystic kidney and hepatic disease). The ultrasonographic appearance of the kidney may be similar to ADPKD but extrarenal (hepatic, pancreatic) cysts are not seen in

ARPKD. Abnormalities in biliary system and hepatic/portal fibrosis or signs of portal hypertension favor the diagnosis of ARPKD.

Autosomal dominant—tuberous sclerosis complex is a rare disease. Patients with tuberous sclerosis can also present with multiple renal cysts associated with renal angiomyolipoma, facial angiofibromas or forehead plaques, ungual or periungual fibroma (small fibromas in or near nails), hypopigmented skin macules called shagreen patch, multiple retinal small nodules (hamartomas).

Autosomal dominant—von Hippel-Lindau disease is syndrome with chances of cancer in many systems. Tumors in eyes, cerebellum, spinal cord, adrenal glands, pancreas, epididymis may be present together with cysts in kidney and pancreas.

Medullary sponge kidney (MSK) is a relatively common disease and usually seen in 4th–5th decades of life. There is defect in the development of medullary pyramids. The region of the renal medulla appears like a sponge due to dilatation of the collecting ducts which are present in the renal medulla. Patients are usually asymptomatic. Stones can form in the dilated collecting ducts and cause hematuria or infections. Presence of small stones within the collecting ducts give an appearance of increased echogenicity of the renal medulla in ultrasonography, bunches of calcification in the medullary region in X-ray (Fig. 17.2) or bunch of grapes

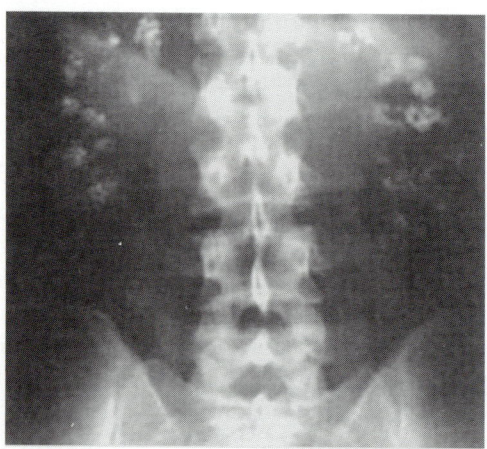

Fig. 17.2: Plain X-ray showing calculi in the renal pyramids in medullary sponge kidney

appearance in intravenous urogram. Patients are usually asymptomatic or have symptoms due to nephrolithiasis, hematuria, or infection. Hypercalciuria may be present. Treatment for hypercalciuria with increased fluid intake, thiazide diuretics. UTI have to be vigorously treated.

LONG-TERM PROGNOSIS IS EXCELLENT

Simple Renal Cysts

These are the commonest acquired cystic lesion and more common in men. They originate from the distal convoluted tubule or collecting ducts and may arise from renal tubular diverticula.

Risk factors for developing such cysts are smoking, increasing age, hypertension and renal dysfunction. They can be unilateral or bilateral; unilocular, single or multiple. They have to be differentiated from ADPKD, RCC or other cystic diseases.

A Bosniak classification can be used to distinguish a simple cyst from complex cyst. This classification is based on USG and CT findings. Thin walls and anechoic contents are indicative of simple cyst, whereas septate thickening and calcification may indicate infection or neoplasia. Thus, cysts with thickened, irregular walls, enhanced septate within the mass are suggestive of complicated cyst. Enhancement of the lesion after intravenous contrast or a multilocular mass may suggest a neoplasia.

Management: Simple cysts are usually left alone. Rarely if pain or hypertension due to compression by a large cyst occurs, USG guided needle drainage can be done. Laparoscopic or retroperitoneoscopic removal of the top of the cyst (cyst de-roofing) is another procedure. Percutaneous drainage can be done if laparoscopic procedure is not available. More complex cysts have to be followed up to find out if they develop signs of malignancy.

18

Hypertension and the Kidney

Reena Thomas, R Kasi Visweswaran

Hypertension is the most common chronic noncommunicable disease in the world. It affects around 25% of the population. The kidney plays a central role in almost all forms of hypertension. It is not only an important cause of hypertension, but also an organ damaged by hypertension. Thus, the kidney can be considered the villain (causing hypertension) and the victim (damaged due to hypertension).

CLASSIFICATION OF HYPERTENSION

According to the latest classification, normal blood pressure means systolic < 120 and diastolic < 80 mm of Hg, prehypertension means systolic 120 to 139 or diastolic 80 to 89 and hypertension means more than 140/90 mm of Hg. Hypertension can be subdivided as Stage (*i*) 140–159/90–99, Stage (*ii*) 160/100 mm. A patient should not be labeled as having hypertension unless: the blood pressure is properly recorded and persistently elevated (even after three to six visits over a several month period or by 24-hour ambulatory monitoring). Hypertension can be either primary when no cause is identified or secondary when an identifiable cause is present (average of 2 or more properly measures readings during two or more visits over a few months observation).

REGULATION OF BLOOD PRESSURE

Blood pressure is the product of cardiac output and peripheral resistance. So, cardiac output and peripheral resistance are the major factors in control of normal and high blood pressure. *Cardiac output* depends on stroke volume and heart rate. *Peripheral resistance* depends on arterioles and smaller blood vessels. The functional and anatomic changes in these blood vessels determine the peripheral resistance (Fig. 18.1). Maintenance of a normal blood pressure is dependent on the balance between the cardiac output and peripheral vascular resistance. Most patients with essential hypertension have a normal cardiac output but a raised peripheral resistance.

Two major systems, the renin angiotensin aldosterone system (RAAS) and the sympathetic nervous system (SNS), regulate the changes in the blood pressure.

Renin Angiotensin Aldosterone System (Fig. 18.2)

Renin is a hormone stored as granules in the modified smooth muscle cells of the afferent arteriole in the juxtaglomerular

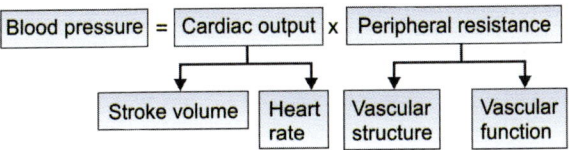

Fig. 18.1: Factors determining blood pressure

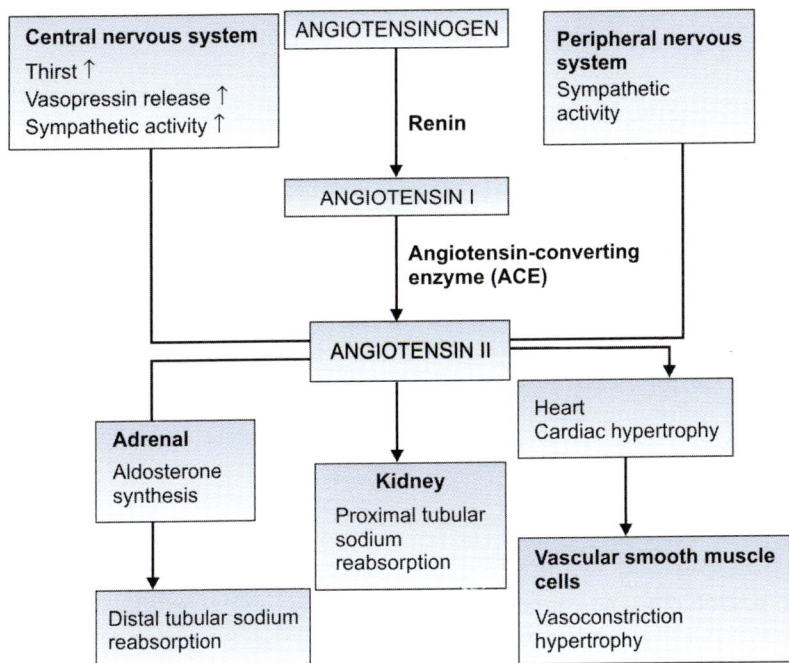

Fig. 18.2: Renin angiotensin aldosterone system

apparatus. It is released to the blood stream in the kidney in response to reduced blood flow to the kidney, reduced salt intake and stimulation of the sympathetic nervous system. This is an important systems that controls blood pressure. Renin converts angiotensinogen (produced from the liver) to angiotensin I. This is converted to angiotensin II (AII) by the angiotensin converting enzyme (ACE). Angiotensin II acts on receptors called AT I receptors and cause vasoconstriction. It also stimulates the hormone aldosterone from the adrenal cortex (zona glomerulosa). Aldosterone causes increase in blood pressure by various mechanisms including:

1. Sodium chloride (salt) retention by the kidney
2. Increased vasoconstriction
3. Decreased vasodilatation (nitric oxide mediated)
4. Increased endothelin production (vasoconstriction)

The renin-angiotensin system may not be directly responsible for the rise in blood pressure in all cases of essential hypertension. Many hypertensive patients, especially elderly and black people may have low levels of renin and angiotensin II. In such instances, drugs that block the RAS are not very effective.

SYMPATHETIC NERVOUS SYSTEM (SNS)

Almost all of the blood vessels except capillaries are supplied by SNS and the stimulation of sympathetic nerves causes vasoconstriction and increase in heart rate. It also causes release of norepinephrine (vasoconstrictor) from the adrenal glands. These factors cause increase in the blood pressure. Moreover, activation of sympathetic nervous system in the kidneys causes decrease in renal blood flow and activation of RAAS. There can be overactivity of the sympathetic nervous system resulting in high blood pressure in the following conditions:

a. Stress and exercise
b. Obesity
c. Insulin resistance
d. Drugs like nicotine, alcohol, cocaine, cyclosporine
e. Defective baroreceptor reflex. (Baroreceptors in the vascular system sense the blood pressure and if there is a change correct it immediately by changes in heart rate.)

PRIMARY OR ESSENTIAL HYPERTENSION

It is the commonest form of hypertension worldwide accounting for nearly 90% of all cases with elevated blood pressure and is defined as blood pressure greater than 140/90 with no identifiable secondary cause.

The pathogenesis is due to many factors and is also decided by the race and hereditary factors. Genetic factors account for about 30% variation in blood pressure. Other causes include low birth weight, reduced number of nephrons in the kidney, or intrauterine developmental disturbances. Abnormalities of genes may determine genetic predisposition (aldosterone synthase gene and adducin gene). African Americans and ethnic minorities like Hispanics have increased chances due to genetic predisposition and obesity. Increased sodium retention by the kidneys and increased sympathetic activity have also been implicated for increasing blood pressure.

With increasing age, thickening and stiffening of arterioles occur. This along with the other factors like diabetes helps to establish persistent hypertension. After a long asymptomatic period, persistent hypertension develops into complicated hypertension. The target organs like kidneys, heart, retina and brain are damaged. The blood vessels, the aorta, and other arteries are also involved.

Risk factors for essential hypertension include:

a. Black race
b. Hypertension in parents
c. Excessive salt intake
d. Obesity, metabolic syndrome
e. Physical inactivity
f. Dyslipidemia,
g. Personality traits

SECONDARY HYPERTENSION

When hypertension results from an underlying identifiable, sometimes correctable cause, it is called secondary hypertension. It accounts for about 10% of all cases of hypertension. The common causes of secondary hypertension and clinical clues are summarized in Table 18.1.

Table 18.1: Medical causes of secondary hypertension

Classification	Examples	Clinical clues
Intrinsic kidney disease	Glomerular disease, e.g. membranoproliferative GN, focal glomerulosclerosis, post-streptococcal GN	Abnormal urinalysis, e.g. proteinuria, hematuria, Red cell casts
	Tubulo-interstitial disease, e.g. polycystic kidney disease acute interstitial nephritis	Elevated creatinine
	Microvascular disease, e.g. thrombotic thrombocytopenic purpura, polyarteritis nodosa, scleroderma.	Abnormal kidney imaging, e.g. multiple cysts
Renovascular disease	Fibromuscular hyperplasia Atherosclerotic renovascular disease	Young age (<40) Abdominal bruit Signs or symptoms of peripheral vascular disease such as claudication, gangrene, TIA, CVA
Mineralocorticoid excess	Primary hyperaldosteronism Cushing syndrome	Hypokalemia Metabolic alkalosis Striae, hirsutism
	Congenital adrenal hyperplasia (11 or 17- hydroxylase deficiency)	Ambiguous genitalia, early puberty (male) or delayed puberty (female)
	Apparent mineralocorticoid excess Glucocorticoid remediable hypertension (familial hyperaldosteronism type I, familial hyperaldosteronism type II)	Family history
Neuroendocrine and neurologic disorders	Pheochromocytoma	Very labile HT episodic flushing, sweating
	Neurofibromatosis	Family history, characteristic physical examination features
Endocrine causes (other)	Hyper/hypothyroidism	Heat/cold intolerance Diarrhea/constipation Weight loss/gain
	Hyperparathyroidism Acromegaly	Kidney stones, bone pain Characteristic physical appearance
	Renin producing tumors	High renin and aldosterone

Contd.

Table 18.1: Medical causes of secondary hypertension (*Contd.*)

Classification	Examples	Clinical clues
Genetic causes	Disorders of sodium homeostatis, e.g. Liddle syndrome, Gordon syndrome polycystic kidney disease	Young age Severe hypertension Family history of kidney disease with abnormal kidney imaging
	Alport's syndrome	Microscopic hematuria, eye changes, sensorineural deafness
Miscellaneous causes	Obesity sleep apnea	Physical examination Excessive snoring, daytime fatigue
	Coarctation of aorta	Discrepancy in PB measurement between arms

Any patient who has clinical clues suggestive of secondary hypertension needs a thorough and extensive evaluation to rule out a secondary cause.

Clues to Presence of Secondary Hypertension

a. Severe or 'resistant' hypertension

b. Sudden increase in blood pressure in a patient with stable control

c. Age <30 years

d. No family history of hypertension

e. Malignant or accelerated hypertension

f. Unexplained deterioration of kidney functions after starting ACE or ARB

g. Severe hypertension in patients with diffuse atherosclerosis.

h. Severe hypertension with asymmetric (>1.5 cm) size of kidneys

i. Flash pulmonary edema

j. Systolic–diastolic abdominal bruit

A few of the secondary causes of hypertension are explained here.

Renal parenchymal hypertension: Renal parenchymal disease is the commonest among the causes of secondary hypertension. In many instances, undetected renal parenchymal disease (IgA nephropathy, focal segmental glomerulosclerosis (FSGS), membranoproliferative GN (MPGN) or other forms of glomerulonephritis) is wrongly labeled as "essential" hypertension. The following are the common renal parenchymal causes:

a. Diabetic nephropathy   40%
b. Hypertensive nephrosclerosis   20%
c. Primary glomerular disease   18%
d. Chronic tubulointerstitial disease   7%
e. Autosomal dominant polycystic kidney disease 5%
f. Obstructive nephropathy   5%

In these cases, hypertension is due to vasoconstricton and salt and water retention.

Control of BP and reduction of proteinuria slow the progression of kidney disease.

The BP should be maintained <140/90 mmHg. ACE inhibitors are main treatment. Diuretics may be added, if necessary. Patient should be monitored for electrolyte anomalies and worsening kidney function.

Renovascular hypertension (RVH): Atherosclerosis and fibromuscular dysplasia are the common causes of RVH. It is due to narrowing of renal arteries or their branches. Atherosclerosis involving the abdominal aorta near the origin of renal arteries may extend to involve the proximal 1/3 of the main renal artery. When it occurs on one side only, it causes unilateral renal artery stenosis. If it involves both sides, it is called bilateral renal artery stenosis. In advanced cases, segmental and diffuse atherosclerosis of intrarenal (inside the kidney) arteries is observed. When involvement is bilateral and diffuse within the kidneys, the condition is called ischemic nephropathy.

a. Ischemic nephropathy is suspected when a patient has azotemia (renal failure) with coronary artery disease, and peripheral vascular disease.

b. Unexplained progressive renal insufficiency in a patient with hypertension

c. Worsening of kidney function after starting ACEi/ARB group of drugs.

d. Occurrence of sudden unexplained "Flash" pulmonary edema.

Fibromuscular dysplasia occurs in females less than 40 years. Here, the structure of the blood vessel is abnormal and results in varying degrees of renal arterial stenosis. Intermittent narrowing by fibrotic bands occurs with aneurysmal dilatation in between. This is due to the absence of internal elastic lamina. This gives rise to 'string of bead' appearance (in angiogram) involving the distal two-thirds of the main renal artery. Based on the vascular layer primarily involved, it is classified into 4 different types:

a. Medial fibroplasia
b. Perimedial fibroplasia
c. Intimal fibroplasia and
d. Adventitial fibroplasia.

If the antihypertensive requirement is less, the condition can be managed by antihypertensive drugs. Procedures like percutaneous transluminal renal angioplasty, renal artery stenting, aortorenal bypass or renal autotransplantation are other procedures undertaken in selected cases.

Resistant hypertension may also be due to renal causes. It is defined as inadequate blood pressure control in a patient adhering to therapeutic doses of 3 antihypertensive agents including a diuretic. It has many causes.

a. Patient not taking medicines as advised
b. Dose of medicines inadequate
c. Choice of medicines incorrect
d. Excessive salt retention (other drugs causing salt retention)
e. Increased sympathetic or RAAS activity.

Renal disease can develop in a patient with essential hypertension when the blood pressure remains uncontrolled for many years. The changes are called benign (hypertensive) nephrosclerosis. In this disorder, long standing hypertension leads to proteinuria and progressive renal failure occur without any other cause.

COMPLICATIONS OF HYPERTENSION

a. *Cardiovascular complications:* Left ventricular hypertrophy, heart failure
b. *Nervous system complications:* Cerebrovascular accidents (Ischemic strokes and cerebral hemorrhage), malignant hypertension and hypertensive encephalopathy.
c. *Kidneys:* Chronic kidney disease (hypertensive nephrosclerosis and malignant hypertension with nephrosclerosis and end stage renal failure) and worsening of other renal diseases.

d. Hypertensive emergency: A condition in which elevated blood pressure results in target organ damage (central nervous system, cardiovascular system, and kidneys). Malignant/accelerated hypertension are hypertensive emergencies. Hypertensive 'emergencies' require immediate therapy to decrease blood pressure.

EVALUATION OF A HYPERTENSIVE PATIENT

The first step is to record blood pressure properly. The blood pressure is recorded first in the right upper limb when the patient is resting and the arm is supported. Blood pressure is recorded by palpation of radial artery first. Next, auscultation at the elbow is done. The sounds heard while the pressure in the cuff are lowered are called 'Korotkoff's sounds'. The first sound is taken as systolic and the muffling is taken as diastolic. During pregnancy, the disappearance of the sounds is the diastolic blood pressure. Ambulatory blood pressure monitoring (ABPM) is a method of recording the blood pressure at periodic intervals for 24 hours by attaching the BP cuff with small electronic equipment to the patient. The data can be fed into a computer and analysed.

The next step will be to find out the extent of target organ damage and risk of target organ damage. Then, curable causes should be looked for and investigations planned later. Presence of family history of hypertension, precipitating factors like use of drugs and secondary causes should also be ruled out.

Evidence of secondary hypertension and target organ damage are looked for in clinical examination. Routine tests consisting of the following are done for all hypertensive patients at the time of diagnosis. They are:

a. Routine urine analysis
b. Hemoglobin/hematocrit,
c. Routine blood chemistries (glucose, blood urea, serum creatinine, serum uric acid, and electrolytes)
d. Estimated glomerular filtration rate (can be calculated from available data)
e. Lipid profile (total and HDL-cholesterol, triglycerides)
f. Electrocardiogram
g. X-ray chest PA view

Additional tests may necessary to rule out secondary causes. These tests are chosen depending on the secondary cause suspected.

STEPS IN TREATMENT

The first step is to contol BP without medicines, if possible. These should be enforced in all prehypertensives and stages 1 and 2 of hypertension. For this, modification of lifestyle is very important. The following are looked into and corrected:

a. Dietary salt restriction
b. Weight loss and regular exercise
c. Decreasing stress factors and adequate sleep
d. Decrease in alcohol intake
e. Stop smoking completely
f. Limit use of NSAIDs and drugs worsening hypertension.

When the patient is already in stage 2 hypertension, simultaneous drug treatment is necessary together with advice on lifestyle modifications. Proper treatment and control of blood pressure reduces the risk of complications. Initially, treatment with one drug (monotherapy) is started. Later, the dose is increased or additional drugs added based on the response. The common drugs used initially are thiazide diuretic, long acting calcium channel blockers or ACE/ARB in uncomplicated hypertension. ACE/ARB are be preferred in diabetics with albuminuria. If a single drug is unable to control the blood pressure well, combination therapy with different drugs help to control the blood pressure. The side effects of the drugs like fluid retention edema, postural hypotension, dry cough, hyperkalemia, worsening of renal failure should be looked for while the patient is on follow up. The patient should be educated not to stop the drugs "because the blood pressure is normal". He must be made to understand that the "normal" blood pressure is because the dose of medicines is correct and he has to continue the same dose otherwise, the blood pressure may worsen.

19

Inherited Disorders of Renal Tubular Function

Jose Paul, R Kasi Visweswaran

The renal tubule forms a part of the nephron and performs many vital functions. The major functions attributed to the renal tubules are:

1. Reabsorption of electrolytes, water, amino acids and glucose that are filtered by the glomerulus. This system is so efficient that nearly 98–99% of the filtrate is reabsorbed, and only 1% is excreted a urine. This process can be adjusted to the body's requirements depending on the environmental conditions, e.g. k if the water intake is more, the tubules help to form more urine and maintain the water balance. If the water intake is less, the tubules reabsorb more water and form lesser volume of urine. Similarly, if the intake of sodium, potassium or other substances is more, the tubules help to excrete them in the urine and if the intake is less, it reabsorbs more and urinary loss is minimized. If the tubules are functioning well, the kidneys can adjust to a wide range of changes, whereas if there is damage to tubules, kidney is unable to maintain the internal environment so effectively.

2. Secretion into urine of certain electrolytes, metabolic products, drugs and toxins, especially protein bound toxins. It helps to eliminate waste products like urea creatinine, uric acid, drugs and toxins.

3. Maintains calcium and phosphate homeostasis by activating vitamin D_3 (cholecalciferol). The inactive cholecalciferol is converted in the liver to 25 hydroxy cholecalciferol. This is converted in the renal tubular cell into its active form called 1,25-dihydroxyvitamin D. In kidney diseases, the active vitamin D is not formed and it leads to bone deformities in children and weakness of bones (osteodystrophy) in adults.

4. Maintains acid–base balance. The proximal tubular cell is concerned mainly with the reabsorption of the bicarbonate ions filtered by the glomerulus and the distal tubular epithelium is concerned with the secretion of hydrogen ions. The hydrogen ions (acid) comes from the food and unless they are excreted, it will neutralize the alkali in the body and result in acidosis. This is why people with renal failure develop acidosis:

Many of the disorders of the renal tubular cell are inherited and include

1. (Inherited) renal tubular acidosis
2. Vitamin D dependant rickets
3. Vitamin D resistant rickets (familial hypophosphatemic rickets —renal phosphate wasting)
4. Bartter's syndrome
5. Gitelman's syndrome
6. Pseudohypoaldosteronism type 1
7. Liddle's syndrome
8. Other disorders of proximal tubular function (cystinuria, Dent's disease, vitamin D dependant rickets).

INHERITED RENAL TUBULAR ACIDOSIS (RTA)

In this group of disorders, the renal tubules are unable to reabsorb bicarbonate that is filtered by the glomerulus and secrete acid (H^+) ions. Secretion of H^+ ions is necessary to remove acid obtained from food and metabolism. Removal of acid ions results in acidification of urine. There are three forms of renal tubular acidosis: Type 1, type 2 and type 3.

Type 1 or Distal RTA

Distal RTA is a defect in the distal tubule. When there is severe metabolic acidosis, the kidney should be able to excrete the H^+ ions and make the urine more acidic. A more acidic urine will have pH of less than 5.5. The other features of distal RTA include hypokalemia, hypocitraturia, hypercalciuria, and nephrocalcinosis. The causes may be inherited or acquired. Inherited causes include mutation of the hydrogen ATPase proton pump (pump responsible for secreting H^+ ions into the tubular lumen) situated in the distal convoluted tubule. This is often associated with sensorineural deafness. The most common cause of acquired distal RTA is

Sjögren's syndrome, a syndrome associated with arthritis and dry conjunctiva and mucous membranes. Treatment is with alkali replacement, 1–3 mmol/kg/day of bicarbonate in divided doses as sodium or potassium citrate. Sodium bicarbonate tablets or Shohl's solution can be used. 1 ml Shohl's solution provides approximately 1 mmol of bicarbonate.

Type 2 or Proximal RTA

This disorder is due to decreased bicarbonate reabsorption in the proximal tubule. The causes may be inherited or acquired. Inherited cause is due to a mutation of the pump for transport of sodium and bicarbonate (cotransporter) in the proximal tubule. Multiple myeloma is a common cause of acquired type 2 RTA. Other acquired causes include drugs, infiltrative disorders, autoimmune disorders and Fanconi's syndrome. Treatment includes identification of any secondary cause and appropriate treatment. Bicarbonate supplements are required at a higher dose of 5–15 mmol/kg/day along with potassium supplementation.

Type 4 RTA

It is associated with hyperkalemia, whereas the other 2 are associated with hypokalemia.

VITAMIN D DEPENDANT RICKETS (VDDR)

There are two types of VDDR, namely type 1 and type 2. Both are inherited as autosomal recessive. Type 1 is due to mutation of the gene which controls the enzyme '1 alpha hydroxylase' which is necessary for conversion of (inactive) 25-hydroxyvitamin D_3 to active 1, 25-dihydroxyvitamin D_3. Type 2 vitamin D dependant rickets is due to end organ resistance to 1, 25-dihydroxyvitamin D_3 due to mutation in the vitamin D receptor. This means that the vitamin D receptor is not able to function and convert 25-hydroxy-vitamin D_3 to active 1, 25-dihydroxyvitamin D_3.

VITAMIN D RESISTANT RICKETS (VDRR)

The disease is inherited as dominant trait and transmitted through the X chromosome. The manifestations are more in the female offsprings. It causes familial hypophosphatemic rickets otherwise known as VDRR. The abnormality is mutation of a gene that controls the formation of fibroblast growth factor 23 (FGF23). This abnormality prevents proper reabsorption of phosphate in the renal tubule. There is loss of phosphates in urine resulting in hypophosphatemia. Phosphates are necessary for bone formation and deficiency causes bony deformities like 'Bow legs'. If phosphate supplements are given by mouth to compensate for the excessive urinary loss, the bone lesions improve and the supplements must be given lifelong.

BARTTER SYNDROME

Bartter syndrome is due to mutations of genes controlling transport of sodium, potassium and chloride in the thick ascending limb of the loop of Henle. There is hypokalemia, alkalosis and the blood pressure is normal even though the renin and aldosterone levels are high. Other features include hypercalciuria and hypomagnesemia. The illness may manifest in the neonatal period or childhood with excessive water drinking (polydipsia) and excessive urination (polyuria). Because of hypercalciuria, kidney stones (nephrocalcinosis) may occur. Renal failure may occur rarely. Liberal fluid, sodium and potassium intake is advised. Drugs like spironolactone (to reduce urinary potassium loss), NSAIDs (to promote sodium retension) and ACE inhibitors (to act against high renin) are sometimes used.

GITELMAN'S SYNDROME

Gitelman's syndrome is due to mutation of genes controlling reabsorption of sodium chloride (NaCl cotransporter) in the distal convoluted tubule. This results in excessive loss of sodium and chloride resulting in hypovolemia and dehydration. Hypomagnesemia and hypocalciuria may also occur. The hypovolemia causes activation of the renin angiotensin aldosterone system leading to hyperaldosteronism. This hyperaldosteronism leads to increased sodium reabsorption in the collecting tubules together with increased potassium and hydrogen ion secretion. Thus, hypokalemia and metabolic alkalosis results. Gitelman's syndrome is more common compared to Bartter syndrome. It presents at a later age with neuromuscular symptoms such as fatigue, weakness, carpo-pedal spasm, tetany, severe hypomagnesemia. These patients need lifelong therapy with potassium and magnesium supplements and liberal salt intake. Spironolactone or amiloride may be used to treat hypokalemia and alkalosis.

PSEUDOHYPOALDOSTERONISM

Aldosterone is a steroid hormone produced from the adrenal cortex. It is important for the control of blood pressure. It causes increase in blood pressure by retaining sodium and excreting potassium. The action of this hormone is mainly in the distal tubule and collecting duct. By retaining sodium and water, it helps to maintain blood pressure. Hypoaldosteronism is decreased aldosterone and may cause hyperkalemia. Pseudohypoaldosteronism (PHA) mimics hypoaldosteronism. If the aldosterone level is not reduced, there is a failure of renal tubuile to respond to the normal aldosterone. There are two independent forms of PHA with different inheritance patterns—(autosomal dominant) renal form with salt loss from the kidneys and (autosomal recessive) multi-system form with salt loss from kidney, lung, and sweat and salivary glands. Treatment of severe forms of PHA is with oral salt supplements and control of hyperkalemia and metabolic acidosis.

LIDDLE'S SYNDROME

This syndrome is due to increased sodium reabsorption by an overactive epithelial sodium channel in the cortical collecting tubule. This disorder closely mimics hyperaldosteronism with hypokalemia, metabolic alkalosis and hypertension. However, plasma aldosterone and renin levels are low due to increased plasma volume. Liddle's syndrome is treated with amiloride which blocks the epithelial sodium channel.

HEREDITARY NEPHROGENIC DIABETES INSIPIDUS

Diabetes insipidus (DI) is a condition due to deficiency of ADH (also called central DI) or due to nonresponsiveness to normal ADH (nephrogenic DI). In nephrogenic DI, although the ADH is secreted by the pituitary gland, the renal tubules fail to respond to it. ADH is also called vasopressin. It is due to mutation of the gene controlling vasopressin 2 receptor in the principal cells of the collecting duct. This results in decreased water reabsorption by the cortical collecting tubule although ADH is present. It usually presents in infancy with polyuria, dehydration, failure to thrive, dilute urine and hypernatremia. Hypernatremia can lead to seizures and mental retardation. It can be treated with liberal water intake along with thiazide diuretics and salt restriction.

20

Diabetes Mellitus and Kidney

R Kasi Visweswaran, Satheesh Balakrishnan

Diabetes mellitus (DM) is a worldwide problem. It is very common in India and the incidence is increasing. Because of the advances in treatment, these patients live longer and have more chances of developing complications of DM. Diabetes can affect the kidney in many ways. Because these patients have atherosclerosis, the blood supply to the kidney may be affected. This can result in hypertension and renal failure. Patients with diabetes are more prone to developing infections. Therefore, infections of the urinary tract are more common in diabetics. After many years, diabetics develop neuropathy. Neuropathy affecting the autonomic nervous system is called autonomic neuropathy. Because of autonomic neuropathy, there can be painless distension of bladder and urinary tract obstruction. Diabetic nephropathy is the commonest microvasculature complication in the kidney. Diabetic nephropathy is also one of the commonest causes of renal failure. More than 40% of patients on maintenance dialysis suffer from advanced stages of diabetic nephropathy. Diabetic nephropathy occurs in both type 1 (known as insulin-dependent or juvenile onset DM) and type 2 (known as noninsulin-dependent or adult onset) DM. Although kidney involvement may be present in a diabetic from the time of diagnosis of DM, it will manifest as diabetic nephropathy clinically only after many years.

Type 2 diabetes is more common than type 1. In both cases, the patients go through a 'silent' stage when all routine investigations will be normal. This stage may last many years. If the control of diabetes is good, the onset of clinical signs of diabetic nephropathy can be delayed by many years. After the silent stage, these patients have a stage called stage of 'persistent microalbuminuria'. During this stage, even though the routine urine examination is normal, the special test for urine albumin by radioimmunoassay will show presence of albumin 30–300 mg/day. The precautions before sending urine sample for microalbuminuria test are

1. Blood sugar must be controlled (FBS ≤110, PPBS ≤180 mg%)
2. Blood pressure must be controlled (BP <140/<90)
3. The urine 'routine' test must be normal
4. At least 2 tests should be done at intervals (3–6 months intervals)
5. Patient should not be suffering from fever or infections
6. Patient should avoid strenuous physical activity (during previous 3 days).

Even during this stage, good control of blood sugar and use of drugs like angiotensin converting enzyme inhibitors to reduce the blood pressure (including blood pressure inside the glomerulus), will protect the kidney from getting damaged quickly. It will be possible to maintain the patient stable for a long time by proper treatment. The next stage is the stage of 'overt clinical nephropathy'. During this stage, the routine urine test for albumin will become positive, hypertension may worsen and these patients develop progressive renal failure. About 10–15% patients will reach end stage renal failure by 20 years from the onset of diabetes and >20% by 30 years.

Patients with long-standing diabetes develop pathologic abnormalities in the kidney. They are:

1. Thickening glomerular basement membrane
2. Sclerosis and expansion of glomerular mesangium
3. Nodules of sclerosis inside the glomeruli (Kimmelstiel-Wilson lesion)
4. Hyaline deposits in the glomerular arterioles
5. Capsular drop
6. Fibrin cap
7. Vacuolisation of tubular cell.

Diabetic nephropathy develops slowly and progress over many years. It begins from a stage of glomerular hypertrophy and hyperfiltration. The hyperfiltration is due to increase in the blood pressure inside the glomeruli. Because of hyperglycemia, the glucose gets bound permanently to all proteins. This is called glycation or glycosylation. When glucose is bound to proteins, the properties of the protein change. These products are called advanced glycation end products (AGE). The AGEs are responsible for mesangial expansion and injury. They also contribute to the development of diabetic nephropathy and other microvascular complications.

Patients with nephropathy usually have other signs of diabetic microvascular disease, such as retinopathy and neuropathy. Retinopathy precedes the onset of overt nephropathy and is easy to detect by ophthalmoscopy. If a patient has features of nephropathy without retinopathy, renal impairment may be part of an independent renal disease.

Diagnosis of diabetic nephropathy is based on the presence of albumin in urine. The usual laborarory test shows proteins in urine. For testing for albumin which is one of the proteins, special tests are necessary. Albustix is the dipstix test for routine testing of albumin. For diagnosing very small quantities of albumin in urine, radioimmunoassay test is necessary. Normal person may excrete less than 30 mg albumin through urine in 24 hours (normoalbuminuria). In microalbuminuria, urinary albumin excretion is between 30 and 299 mg/24 hrs. During this stage testing by radioimmunoassay will be necessary for diagnosis. If urinary albumin excretion is more than 300 mg/24 hours, it is called clinical (overt) albuminuria. To diagnose this stage, simple albustix test is sufficient. Diabetic patients are advised to check the urine periodically. Abnormal urinary albumin excretion suggests development of nephropathy. If albuminuria is present for more than 3 months, chronic kidney disease (CKD) can be confirmed. The severity of renal involvement can be staged as per estimated creatinine clearance (eGFR) (please see chapter on CKD for detailed classification). The staging of CKD as per eGFR is shown in Table 20.1.

Table 20.1: Stages of CKD based on eGFR

CKD stage	eGFR level (ml/min/1.73 m^2)
Stage 1	≥90
Stage 2	60–89
Stage 3	30–59
Stage 4	15–29
Stage 5	<15

Initially, the patient may not have any symptoms. When the kidney functions are reduced, the patient may develop hypertension and edema. When a diabetic patient develops hypoglycemia frequently while he is using the same earlier dose of medicines, onset of renal failure should be suspected. Normally, >50% of insulin is degraded by the kidneys. When the kidneys fail, they do not degrade the insulin. So, it may cause hypoglycemia. When the kidney functions worsen to stage 4 or 5, it will be necessary to plan a vascular access and prepare for dialysis. It is also possible for them to undergo renal transplantation.

The treatment should aim to slow the progression of kidney damage and control related complications. From the early stages, good control of blood sugar will help to prevent or delay the complications by many years. The aim should be to keep the blood sugar continuously within the normal range. Oral antidiabetic drugs or insulin can be used as required. When microalbuminuria occurs, the main treatment is using angiotensin converting enzyme inhibitor (ACEi) drugs or angiotensin receptor blocking drugs (ARBs) which help to reduce proteinuria and slow the progression of diabetic nephropathy. The renal protection is due to the antihypertensive effect, renal vasodilatation, improved renal blood flow and dilatation of the efferent arterioles. The main side effects are dry cough and hyperkalemia. Diet may be modified to help control blood sugar levels. Modification of protein intake is useful and is advised only in those who use high quantities of red meat. Blood pressure should be well controlled with antihypertensive medications, in order to reduce the risks of kidney, eye, heart and brain. It is also very important to control lipid levels, maintain a healthy weight, and engage in regular physical activity. Patients with diabetic nephropathy should avoid using nephrotoxic drugs like radio contrast agents, non-steroidal anti-inflammatory drugs (NSAIDs) and aminoglycosides, because they may injure the weakened kidney. Infections should be treated with appropriate antibiotics.

When the renal function worsens, early planning for dialysis should be done. In patients with diabetes, there may be vascular disease and so the vascular access may not develop satisfactorily. Kidney transplantation can also be performed in diabetics on dialysis due to CKD stage 5. In type 1 diabetes, combined kidney and pancreatic islet cell (kidney pancreas) transplantation is advisable. Diabetic nephropathy is a progressive disease. Complications due to renal failure occur earlier and progress more rapidly in diabetics when compared to nondiabetics. People with diabetes do worse than nondiabetics on dialysis or after renal transplantation. Therefore, the best strategy should be to strictly control diabetes from the very early stages and periodically check for proteinuria, blood pressure and kidney function.

21

Systemic Lupus Erythematosus and Kidney

Manu G Krishnan, R Kasi Visweswaran

Systemic lupus erythematosus (SLE) is a multisystem disease usually associated with exacerbations (flares) and remissions (quiescence). It is more common in young females. It is due to production of antibodies (Abs) to own cells or tissues. Such Abs are called autoantibodies. In systemic lupus erythematosus, there is an inappropriate response of the immune system against the cells in the body. There are 2 types of autoimmune diseases:

a. Organ specific (antibodies against a specific organ or gland) **Example:** Thyroid gland

b. Systemic (antibodies against many antigens involving many organs and tissues)

SLE is characterised by inflammation in multiple organs, blood vessels, and other connective tissues in the body. Tissue damage occurs as a result of cell mediated immune responses and direct damage by autoantibodies or immune complexes. Autoantibodies (Ab) found in SLE may be against the nuclei known as antinuclear Ab (ANA), against double stranded DNA (anti-dsDNA Ab), or against phospholipid known as antiphospholipid Ab (APLA). Antibodies are formed against histones, RBCs, platelets, leukocytes and clotting factors. Ab against RBCs and platelets can lead to complement-mediated lysis resulting in anemia and thrombocytopenia. Presence of APLA is associated with thrombotic tendency and repeated abortions.

ETIOLOGY

a. **Genetic factors:** Genetic factors predispose an individual to have this disease. If one of the identical twins is suffering from SLE, the chances in the other twin increases 10 times. 10% of individuals with SLE may have a family member affected by the same disease. Genes that control the predisposition to have SLE are not completely understood now.

b. **Environmental factors:** It is more common in African American women, Spanish and Indian women compared to the white race (Caucasians).

c. **Hormonal factors:** Women are 10 times more likely than men to get this disease. Female hormone particularly estrogen may be responsible for higher incidence in young women.

d. **Other factors:** Exposure to ultraviolet light, smoking, physical and emotional stress, drugs and infections are other important etiological factors.

PATHOGENESIS

SLE is an immune complex disease where antigens and antibodies combine together to form immune complexes and are deposited in various parts of the body. Since the antigens (Ag) are body's own proteins, the antibodies are called autoantibodies and belong to immunoglobulin G (IgG) type. When immune complexes are deposited in tissues, they activate the complement system in the blood. Various mediators of inflammation are released from the site of Ag-Ab deposition. Thus, acute inflammatory reaction occurs.

The body proteins which may become antigenic in SLE are:

a. Nuclei — anti-nuclear Ab (ANA)

b. DNA — anti-dsDNA (anti-dsDNA Ab)

c. Cardiolipin (phospholipid) — anticardiolipin antiphospholipid Ab (APLA)

d. Smooth muscle — anti-Sm

e. Histone — antihistone

ANA can be positive in other conditions also. Anti-dsDNA is more specific and seen in lupus nephritis, APLA is associated with thrombosis and recurrent abortions, anti-Sm is highly specific for SLE and antihistone is more common in drug-induced lupus.

CLINICAL FEATURES

Symptoms are extremely variable. In SLE, fever, weight loss, rash (butterfly rash), hairloss, oral ulceration, central nervous system involvement, renal involvement, joint pain/arthritis or arthralgia, liver disorders, serositis and blood disorders may occur. Most of the symptoms of this disease result from the deposition of immune complexes within various tissues followed by local type III hypersensitivity reaction. The American College of Rheumatology has suggested that 4 or more of the criteria given below must be present for diagnosing SLE (Table 21.1).

Renal involvement occurs in more than 80% of patients with SLE. Changes in renal biopsy in SLE includes vascular, glomerular and tubule-interstitial changes. Based on renal histology SLE is divided as class 1 to class 6. This classification is useful for deciding the prognosis and treatment. In SLE all types of immunoglobulins will be seen in the biopsy under immunofluorescent microscopy.

DIAGNOSIS

The clinical manifestations and presence of serologic markers (autoantibodies) help to confirm SLE. Urine analysis for proteinuria and microscopy are important for identifying renal involvement. Proteinuria is usually present. Urine deposits may show various cellular elements and casts. This appearance in urine is called 'telescoped urinary sediment'. The blood examination often shows anemia, leucopenia and thrombocytopenia. Serum ANA is elevated in more than 90% and is highly sensitive screening test for SLE patients. Autoantibodies against dsDNA are more specific and are present in about three-fourths of untreated lupus patients. The ELISA is the most commonly used assay. Sm antibodies are highly specific for lupus nephritis but may be present only in about 25% to 30% of patients. Antibodies to C1q (anti-C1q Ab) are more closely associated with the activity. So, they have a prognostic role

Table 21.1: American College of Rheumatology criteria for diagnosis of SLE

1. Malar rash
2. Discoid rash
3. Photosensitivity
4. Oral ulcers
5. Arthritis   (non-erosive arthritis)
6. Serositis   (pleuritis, pericarditis)
7. Renal disease   (proteinuria, cellular casts)
8. Neurologic disorder   (seizures, psychosis)
9. Hematologic disorder (anemia, leucopenia and thrombocytopenia)
10. Positive immunologic tests (increased anti-dsDNA Ab, anti-Sm Ab)
11. Positive fluorescent antinuclear Ab.

in the follow-up of patients with lupus nephritis. Serum levels of total hemolytic complement and complement components C3 and C4 are often depressed in active lupus. Assessment of disease activity is important in the treatment of SLE. Proteinuria, 'active' urinary sediment (microscopic hematuria with various types of cells and casts), anemia, leucopenia, thrombocytopenia, rising anti-dsDNA antibody titre, low complement are suggestive of disease activity.

TREATMENT

Prevention is by avoiding exposure to sunlight (ultraviolet rays), prevention of infection and avoidance of smoking. Treatment is given to improve the symptoms and diminish the activity of the disease. Long-term treatment and follow-up are essential and complete cure may not be possible in most cases. The treatment chosen depends on clinical manifestations and biopsy findings. More powerful drugs are used for more severe disease activity. Those with no renal involvement are given hydroxychloroquin, non-steroidal anti-inflammatory drugs (NSAIDs) and small doses of prednisolone. Those with renal involvement are given prednisolone and other immunosuppressive drugs like cyclophosphamide, azathioprine, or mycophenolate initially. Immunosuppressive drugs help by slowing proliferation of antibody producing cells. Procedures like plasmaphresis are done to remove the antibodies in very severe cases. The treatment is continued till the patient is in remission and the patient is closely followed up thereafter.

With systematic treatment and follow up, the prognosis of SLE has improved significantly over the last few decades. The patient and their families should be counseled on proper diet, rest, exercise, avoidance of exposure to UV light, smoking and the need for regular follow-up.

22

Pregnancy and the Kidney

R Kasi Visweswaran

Pregnancy is physiological and is associated with a number of changes in the anatomy and physiology of the mother. These changes help the embryo to develop so that the mother can deliver a healthy baby. The important changes that occur in both kidneys and urinary tract are increase in the size by 1 cm, weight and volume by 30%. These changes disappear within a few weeks of delivery of the child.

The pelvicalyceal system and ureters undergo dilation. The dilation is more on the right side and the ureteric dilation is usually up to the pelvic brim. Since there is increased cardiac output by 30–40%, the renal blood flow and glomerular filtration rate (GFR) are also increased. The increase in GFR starts soon after conception and persists till delivery. Because of this, the level of blood urea, serum creatinine and serum uric acid are lower compared to non-pregnant state. The normal limits of renal functions during pregnancy are given below.

Blood urea	=	20–27 mg/dl
Or BUN	=	10–13 mg/dl
Serum creatinine	=	0.7–0.9 mg/dl
Serum uric acid	=	2.5–4.0 mg/dl

Even though the blood volume and cardiac output are high during pregnancy, the blood pressure decreases compared to non-pregnant level. The blood pressure decreases from the time of conception gradually to reach the lowest systolic and diastolic BP by the end of 2nd trimester. During the 3rd trimester it gradually increases and by the time of delivery, it reaches the original (pre-pregnant) levels (Fig. 22.1).

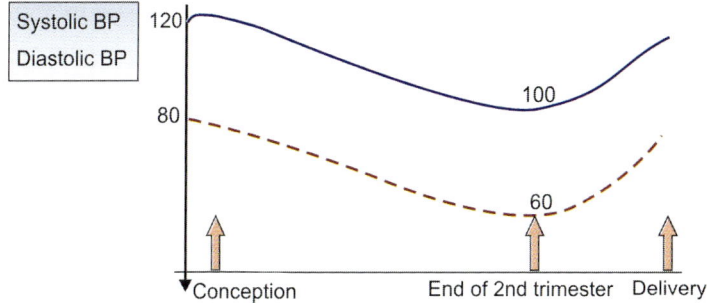

Fig. 22.1: Blood pressure changes in normal pregnancy

The criteria for diagnosis of hypertension in pregnant women are:

1. Systolic BP >140
2. Diastolic BP >90

One high recording does not confirm the diagnosis unless the value is over 160/100. There must be 2 values with at least 6 hours gap between them to confirm the diagnosis if BP is >140/90 and less than 160/100. The hypertensive disorders in pregnancy can be classified as follows:

1. Pre-eclampsia/eclampsia
2. Chronic hypertension (pre-existing)
3. Superimposed pre-eclampsia
4. Late transient hypertension

PRE-ECLAMPSIA/ECLAMPSIA

Pre-eclampsia is a type of hypertension which occurs during pregnancy. It is usually associated with proteinuria, edema, and abnormal weight gain which occur after 20th week of gestation. It is more common in primigranida, teenage pregnancies, pregnancy after 35 years, multiple pregnancies, mothers with diabetes, vesicular mole, fetal anomalies or polyhydramnios. The blood pressures during early pregnancy will be normal and the BP increases only after 20th week. There may be increase in hemoglobin and hematocrit. The platelet count may be low and the liver enzymes may be elevated. HELLP (hypertension elevated liver enzymes low platelets count) syndrome is a type of severe pre-eclampsia. When convulsion occurs, it is called eclampsia. The blood pressure returns to normal soon after delivery. Low dose aspirin and high dose of oral calcium carbonate are used to prevent the occurrence of PIH.

CHRONIC HYPERTENSION

Hypertension in pregnancy may be due to pre-existing the undiagnosed hypertension detected for the first time during pregnancy. This occurs because the BP may be checked for the first time only during pregnancy. In these women also, the BP will decrease from the original level till end of the second trimester.

SUPERIMPOSED PRE-ECLAMPSIA

Patients with chronic hypertension have higher chances of developing pre-eclampsia or eclampsia. So, the patients must be treated with drugs to bring down the BP to normal levels. This will reduce the risks to the mother and fetus.

LATE TRANSIENT HYPERTENSION

In late transient hypertension, the BP increases in late pregnancy towards labor and the blood pressure settles down to normal shortly after delivery. This is not usually associated with proteinuria.

High blood pressure in the mother is harmful for the fetal growth and development. Therefore, antihypertensive drugs are used to keep the BP in the normal range for pregnancy. Intrauterine growth retardation or even intrauterine death may occur in women with uncontrolled hypertension during pregnancy. Antihypertensive drugs like alpha methyl dopa, hydralazine, Labetolol and some calcium channel blocking drugs can be used safely during pregnancy. Drugs like angiotensin converting enzyme inhibitors, angiotensin receptor blockers, most of the beta blockers (propranolol group) are avoided during pregnancy.

Urinary tract infection during pregnancy is common. It may be asymptomatic bacteruria, symptomatic lower urinary infection or pyelonephritis. Any infection should be promptly treated. Asymptomatic bacteruria is characterised by positive urine cultures in an asymptomatic women during pregnancy. Untreated asymptomatic bacteruria is associated with increased risk of hypertension, premature delivery, anemia and low birth weight babies. Lower urinary infections may be recurrent and it may be necessary to give low dose long-term antibiotics. Although acute pyelonephritis is rare, it may lead to sepsis, shock, renal abscess or renal failure. Hence, these patients require hospitalization and parenteral antibiotics. Aminoglycosides, quinolones are avoided during pregnancy.

Acute kidney injury may occur in early pregnancy due to septic abortion, dehydration and severe morning sickness (hyperemesis gravidarum). During late pregnancy, the causes of acute kidney injury are:

a. Abruptio placentae and severe bleeding
b. Uncontrolled severe hypertension
c. Acute fatty liver of pregnancy
d. Idiopathic postpartum acute renal failure
e. Postpartum hemorrhage-disseminated intravascular coagulation (DIC).

The renal tubules undergo necrosis and the patient may need dialysis till recovery occurs. Rarely the tubules, in the renal cortex, may be severely affected leading to 'cortical necrosis'. These patients will require long-term dialysis or even renal transplantation.

Conditions like nephrotic syndrome, chronic nephritis, IqA nephropathy, SLE may be associated with higher chances for developing hypertension or intrauterine growth retardation. Some illness like MPGN may worsen during pregnancy. SLE usually worsens toward term or after delivery and the dose of immunosuppressive drugs is increased after delivery. In all these cases if the hypertension is controlled well and renal failure is absent, the outcome of pregnancy is favorable.

23

Drugs and Kidney

R Kasi Visweswaran, Manu G Krishnan

Drugs are chemical compounds used for prevention, diagnosis or treatment of various diseases. Every drug has some actions on the body. The drug is absorbed, distributed to various parts of the body where they act. They are metabolized and excreted from the body. The kidney is the major organ through which many of the drugs are excreted. The term pharmacodynamics means the actions of the drug or "what the drug does to the body". The term pharmacokinetics means "what the body does to the drugs" which means how the body absorbs, distributes, metabolises and excretes the drug.

VULNERABILITY OF KIDNEYS: WHY THE KIDNEYS ARE AFFECTED BY DRUGS

The kidneys are easily affected by drugs or toxic substances because of the following reasons:

a. Although the kidneys weigh only 300 gm, i.e. 0.5% of body wt, they get 25–30% of cardiac output. Thus, the blood supply is very high 3.5–4.0 ml/gm of renal tissue. This is the organ having highest blood supply/gm of tissue. Brain tissue and liver get only 1 ml/gm of tissue. Therefore, large quantities of drugs/toxins reach the kidney every minute.

b. If the drug or toxin is filtered by the glomerulus, the concentration of the drug will increase further in the filtrate. If it is not filtered, it will reach the peritubular capillaries in a high concentration. Drugs with a molecular weight of less than 60,000 Daltons are freely filtered through the glomerulus. Lipid soluble substances (non-polar) drugs diffuse readily across tubular cells, whereas water soluble compounds (polar) do not. Since most drugs are excreted by the kidneys, they can be damaged more easily compared to other organs.

c. If the filtered drug/toxin remains in tubular fluid without being reabsorbed, it reaches very high concentration because most of the water is reabsorbed.

d. If the filtered drug is reabsorbed by the tubule cell, it will reach inside the tubule cell in high concentration.

e. The tubular cells have high metabolic and enzymatic activity. This makes the kidneys highly susceptible to injury because the drugs can interfere with the metabolism and enzymatic activity. Use of multiple drugs cause more damage due to toxic action in different parts of the kidney. Drugs are a very common cause of acute kidney injury and chronic kidney disease.

f. Since all natural products are also chemical compounds, they can also cause kidney damage.

g. Drugs can alter the blood circulation in the kidney or damage the endothelial lining of the blood vessel or capillaries causing damage.

MECHANISM OF KIDNEY DAMAGE (NEPHROTOXICITY) DUE TO DRUGS

The damage to the kidney can be more if the dose of the toxic drug is very high. Older individuals have lesser kidney function. So they are at higher risk. In infants and premature babies, the kidneys may not be fully developed. Therefore, they are at higher risk. If the patient has other medical conditions like hypotension, hypokalemia, hypomagnesemia, sepsis, coma, convulsions, muscle damage, liver damage, hypoalbuminemia or when there is pre-existing renal damage, the chance of nephrotoxicity will be higher. The damage can be more when 2 or more nephrotoxic drugs are given at the same time. The duration of administration is also important. Some drugs may cause kidney damage because of allergic/anaphylactic reaction. Some drugs cause alteration in the blood supply to the kidney and cause damage. This is called hemodynamically mediated renal damage.

Four important drugs commonly used in the hospitals which cause nephrotoxicity are discussed briefly. Aminoglycoside group of antibiotics, angiotensin converting enzyme inhibitor group, nonsteroidal anti-inflammatory drugs and radiocontrast media are the 4 important group of drugs causing nephrotoxicity. Many other drugs also cause nephrotoxicity.

AMINOGLYCOSIDE GROUP OF ANTIBIOTICS

Aminoglycosides group of antibiotics like gentamycin, kanamycin, tobramycin or amikacin are used in the treatment of Gram- negative infections. The drug accumulates in the proximal convoluted tubule and affects its functioning leading to acute kidney injury and renal failure. The damage to renal tubule and the toxicity is usually related to the total dose (dose + duration of use). A high index of suspicious is necessary for early diagnosis, because in the early stages the urine output may be normal although there is progressive increase in urea and creatinine. This condition is called 'non-oliguric acute renal failure'. Since the drug accumulates in the renal tubule, cumulative toxicity may occur and the duration of renal failure may be greatly prolonged. Aminoglycoside nephrotoxicity can be prevented by:

1. Careful use in all patients especially high-risk cases
2. Dose reduction in patients with renal dysfunction
3. Maintaining adequate hydration and urine output
4. Avoiding use of other nephrotoxic drugs.

Since aminoglycosides are removed by dialysis, loading dose of the drug should be given after each dialysis to maintain the blood level sufficient for its action. This blood level is also called 'therapeutic window'.

NONSTEROIDAL ANTI-INFLAMMATORY DRUGS (NSAIDs)

NSAIDs cause renal damage by causing nephritic syndrome, salt and water tension, renal papillary necrosis, hyperalkaline and suppression of renal autoregulation. Elderly persons who have dehydration, pre-existing renal disease, those who consume other nephrotoxic drugs or are more prone to renal injury due to NSAIDs.

The clinical features are fluid retention, oliguria and increase in blood urea and serum creatinine. NSAIDs cause renal failure in different ways. It affects older persons those with dehydration, underlying renal diseases, kidney/heart/liver failure or when used with other drugs capable of damaging the kidney. In addition to oliguria and acute kidney injury, they may also cause nephrotic syndrome and hyperkalemia. Long-term steady use of analgesics like acetaminophen may cause renal papillary necrosis. In view of such deadly complications, it is necessary to use NSAIDs very carefully and observe the patient closely.

RADIOCONTRAST AGENTS

Radiocontrast agents are iodine containing dyes used to visualize parts of the body more clearly in the X-ray. In view of its usefulness as a diagnostic and therapeutic tool, it is used extensively in clinical practice. The earlier radiocontrast agents were 'ionic' and 'hyperosmolar' and caused renal toxicity. The modern radiocontrast agents are 'nontoxic' and 'iso-osmolar' and so, they cause lesser toxicity. However, since the use and doses have increased contrast induced acute kidney injury is the one of the commonest causes of AKI in hospitalized patients. The onset of renal problem is within 24–48 hrs of exposure to radiocontrast. Usually patients develop oliguria associated with worsening of renal function.

The risk factors are the same as in NSAID induced damage. In addition, the use of 'ionic' contrast media, larger dose intra-arterial use and repeated use are associated with higher chances of kidney damage. It can be prevented to some extent by careful use, minimum dose, maintaining good hydration and good urine output.

Use of drugs to alkalinize the urine and drugs like N-acetylcysteine or fenoldepam are used occasionally. If progressive renal failure occurs, dialysis support may be necessary.

Angiotensin Converting Enzymes—Inhibitors/Angiotensin Receptor Blockers

These drugs are used increasingly in the treatment of hypertension, cardiac disease and diabetic nephropathy. Although they are very useful, they may cause complication like worsening of renal failure, hyperkalemia and dry cough. Angiostensin II is necessary for autoregulation of normal circulation. The autoregulation helps to keep the pressure in the glomerular capillaries sufficient enough to result in glomerular filtration. The angiostensin II does this by increasing the tone of the efferent glomerular artery. When angiostensin is not produced because of the use of angiostensin converting enzyme, inhibitor drugs or when angiostensin II action is blocked by A_2 receptor blocking drugs, this protection (autoregulation) is lost and the glomerular filtration is reduced. Therefore, these drugs are used carefully by monitoring serum creatinine and serum potassium.

Prescribing Drugs in Renal Failure

Before starting treatment with a known nephrotoxic drug, it is necessary to assess the renal function by calculating creatinine clearance. The simplest bedside formula for calculation in adults is Cockroft-Gault formula.

$$\text{Creatinine clearance} = \frac{\{140 - age\ (years)\} \times wt(kg)}{72 \times serum\ creatinine\ (mg\%)} \times (0.85 \text{ for females})$$

For proper administration of drugs in a patient with renal disease, 3 steps are necessary.

1. *Choosing a loading dose:* The loading dose is usually similar to a patient with normal renal function. The maintenance dose is adjusted according to the degree of renal function as assessed by eGFR.

2. *Choose a maintenance dose:* The maintenance dose can be given by reducing the dose each time or changing the dosing interval. Dose adjustment is usually not required when the CrCl is >50 ml/min.

   Dosing interval can be changed depending on the following calculation. It may be different for different drugs.

$$\text{Dosing interval} = \frac{\text{Normal creatinine} \times \text{normal interval}}{\text{Patient's creatinine}}$$

(Varying interval method may lead to subtherapeutic drug concentration in between)

Maintenance dose = Patient's creatinine × normal dose

3. *Perform therapeutic drug monitoring (TDM):* It is possible to do TDM for only some drugs.

Careful use of drugs, appropriate dose modifications depending on age, the level of renal function and avoidance of such drugs in high-risk individuals help a lot in reducing drug-induced renal failure.

24

Dialysis and Related Procedures

Jose Paul, R Kasi Visweswaran

The word 'dialysis' is from Greek terms—*dia* means 'through' and *lysis* means 'separate and remove'. Dialysis is a life-saving procedure done when the kidneys fail. The waste products which are normally excreted by the kidneys accumulate in the body in renal failure. Dialysis helps to remove some of the waste products and maintain the internal environment. There are mainly 2 types of dialysis, peritoneal dialysis and hemodialysis. The principles involved in dialysis are osmosis, diffusion and ultrafiltration. Dialysis when two solutions are separated by a semipermeable membrane, substances move across the membrane depending on whether the membrane permits the substance to pass through. A solution contains solute (solid) which is dissolved in the solvent (liquid). In sugar solution, sugar is the solute and water is the solvent.

If 2 solutions with different solute concentrations are separated by a semipermeable membrane, the solvent (liquid) moves from the side of lower solute concentration to the side of higher solute concentration. This is called osmosis.

In diffusion, there is movement of solute from the side of higher solute concentration to the side of lower (solute) concentration if the membrane is permeable to the specific solutes.

Ultrafiltration is the movement of the solvent across the membrane from an area of higher to lower hydrostatic pressure. Most types of dialysis use one or more of the above principles.

Solvent drag is the name given to the process in which, the fast movement of the solvent across the membrane drags or transports more solutes along with it. Thus, the solute movement also increases.

PERITONEAL DIALYSIS

In peritoneal dialysis, the normal lining in the abdomen called peritoneum is used as the semipermeable membrane for filtering the blood. A sterile dialysis solution which has electrolyte concentration similar to plasma is instilled into the peritoneal cavity by gravity, undertaking all sterile precautions. When the fluid remains in the peritoneal cavity, it is separated from the blood by the peritoneal (semipermeable) membrane. Waste products in the blood will diffuse from the blood to the fluid. Water will also move from blood to the fluid by osmosis. The electrolytes can move either way depending on the concentration gradient. After some time (dwell time) the fluid is drained and replaced with fresh fluid (Fig. 24.1). Each such procedures is called a 'cycle'. The quantity of sterile dialysis fluid used for dialysis is about 2 litres for adult and 50 ml/kg body weight in children. Many 'cycles' or exchanges are performed. Absolute sterile precautions are necessary. Air should not be allowed to enter the dialysis tubings and the system is operated using only the external cramps.

There are 3 types of peritoneal dialysis:
1. Continuous ambulating peritoneal dialysis (CAPD)
2. Continuous cyclic peritoneal dialysis
3. Intermittent peritoneal dialysis

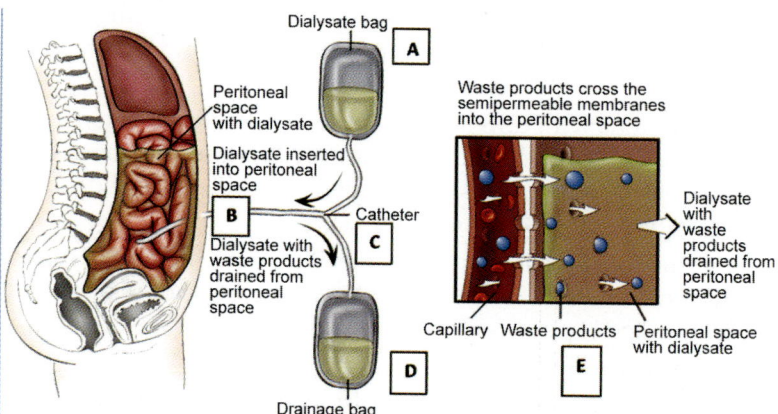

Fig. 24.1: Peritoneal dialysis. Note: Dialysate bag (A), peritoneal catheter in the peritoneal cavity (B), Y connection helping drainage of dialysis fluid by gravity (C) and drainage bag (D). The inset shows movement on molecules across the peritoneal membrane (E).

CONTINUOUS AMBULATING PERITONEAL DIALYSIS (CAPD)

In this type, the patient or attendant is trained to perform the exchanges. There is no machine. The bags with the solution and tubings are specially suited for self use at home. The dwell time is long—usually 4–6 hrs. The procedure is continuous. During the 'dwell time' the patient is able to do normal activities. Three or four exchanges are performed every day depending on the prescription and each exchange may take 30–40 minutes. One end of the dialysis catheter with small holes is placed in the peritoneal cavity and the other end is taken out through a subcutaneous tunnel through the anterior abdominal wall. The subcutaneous portion of the catheter has usually 2 cuffs which help to fix the catheter in position and prevent infection from reaching the peritoneum through the outside of the catheter. Clean technique is taught to the patient to prevent introduction of infection through the catheter.

The patient is trained to maintain a chart showing "fluid in", "fluid out", daily weight urine output. This helps in deciding the amount of oral fluid intake. Since proteins are lost from the body through the peritoneal dialysis fluid drained from the body, the patient should be given a high protein diet (about 2.5–3 gm/kg/day). The patient must be monitored for dialysis efficiency, ability to remove fluid from the body, status of nutrition and evidence of infection by periodic check up. The patient must have adequate bowel movement and should not be constipated for successful functioning of CAPD exchanges. Although the fluid and connecting tubes are expensive, it is ideal method of treatment for

a. Very old patients—they will find it difficult to travel to dialysis centre 2–3 times a week.
b. Those with hepatitis B/C (high chance of spread of infection to staff and other patients in hemodialysis). If totally separate isolation dialysis facility is available, hemodialysis may be considered.
c. As temporary dialysis before renal transplantation.
d. In children—the timings can be adjusted so that the child can attend school.

CONTINUOUS (NOCTURNAL) CYCLER (ASSISTED) PERITONEAL DIALYSIS

In this types of dialysis, the patient connects himself to a compact machine called peritoneal dialysis cycler before going to bed. The cycler will perform the peritoneal dialysis cycles during the night.

The patient can be disconnected from the cycler after 8–10 hrs. He will have to repeat this every night. He can pursue his regular work during daytime.

Intermittent Peritoneal Dialysis

Intermittent PD is done in the hospital as a temporary measure or for acute kidney injury. The dwell time is short (30 minutes) and approximately, one exchange can be completed in one hour. Each session of IPD requires 40 litre exchanges (20 exchanges of 2 L each). Two or three sessions will be required every week. IPD cannot be continued for a long time. Sterile precautions should be strictly followed.

HEMODIALYSIS

When hemodialysis was invented after the Second World War in late 1940s, the equipment was large and crude. It consisted of a rotating drum, a tank of electrolyte solution, cellphone membranes and plastic tubings. Today, the machines are electronically controlled with numerous safety systems and hemodialysis has now become a relatively simple and painless procedure. Three important requirements are necessary for hemodialysis:

1. Vascular access
2. Artificial kidney
3. Hemodialysis machine (monitor)

Vascular Access

Vascular access is an arrangement by which blood can be taken out of the body at the rate of about 250–300 ml/minute and returned after dialysis. The blood flows outside the body through tubes to the artificial kidney and back to the patient. The part of the blood flow outside the body is called 'extracorporeal blood circuit'. The vascular access may be temporary or permanent. Temporary vascular access is through dialysis catheters—single lumen or double dialysis lumen catheter. If a single lumen catheter can be placed in a larger vein like femoral or jugular vein, and another suitable subcutaneous vein canulated with a large bore fistula needle, it can be used as a temporary vascular access. In double lumen dialysis catheters, there are 2 lumens inside the catheter. Each lumen has a separate external opening through a connector. One lumen is used to take blood from the patient and the other lumen to return the blood.

Arteriovenous shunt (Scribner shunt): This was one of the earliest successful vascular accesses used in patients for over quarter century. The radial artery is canulated above the wrist using a teflon vessel tip which is connected to a silastic catheter. The cephalic vein in the forearm is also canulated similarly. The 2 silastic connecting tubes can be connected to each other or separated. During dialysis, the 2 tubes are separated and connected to the 2 limbs of the extracorporeal circuit. After dialysis they are reconnected to each other till the next dialysis. The vessel tip remains inside the body but the silastic tube remains outside the body covered by protective bandage. AV shunt is no longer used.

The most effective and preferred permanent access is a arteriovenous fistula in the forearm. This fistula is called Brescia-Cimeno fistula. For this a suitable artery and vein should be close to each other so that they can be interconnected. When an internal communication is created surgically between radial artery and cephalic vein in the lower forearm, the blood from the radial artery flows directly to the cephalic vein. The wall of the vein becomes thicker and blood flow through the vein increases. In about 6–8 weeks, the vein enlarges, develops a thick wall and has high rate of blood flow. This is called maturing of the fistula (Fig. 24.2). When mature, these enlarged and thick walled veins can be punctured with a large bore needle to obtain sufficient blood flow for dialysis. These large bore needles with extension tube suitable for connecting with the extracorporeal circuit are called 'fistula needles' (Fig. 24.3). They are disposable single use needles. Since there is no foreign tissue, it remains functional for many years. If the artery and veins in the forearm are not suitable, brachial artery can be connected with the cephalic vein and the brachiocephalic AV fistula allowed time for maturing before use.

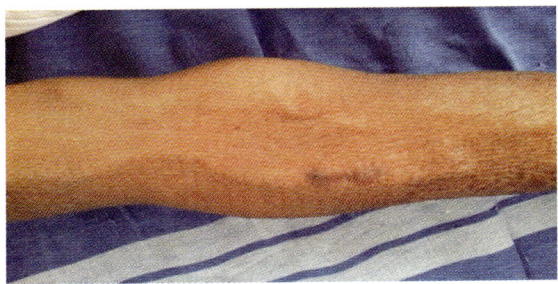

Fig. 24.2: AV fistula. Please note the enlarged superficial veins

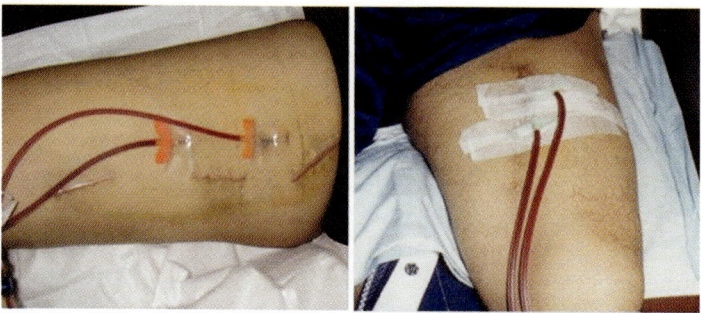

Fig. 24.3: AV fistula cannulated with fistula needles for dialysis

'In rare situations when suitable artery and vein are not available close by, it may be necessary to introduce a segment of vein from other parts of the body or synthetic tubes to connect the artery and vein. This is called an AV graft. Saphenous vein harvested from the leg of the same individual or synthetic grafts are used. The synthetic graft is made of polytetrafluoroethylene (PTFE). They can be connected between radial artery at the wrist to cephalic vein at the elbow. Here, the graft will be straight and the blood flow will be from wrist towards elbow. If the brachial artery and cephalic vein are connected at the elbow, the graft is taken through a loop in the forearm under the skin (Fig. 24.4). The part of the loop near the artery can be punctured to take the blood away from the body and the part near the cephalic vein used to return the blood.

Permanent access can be achieved using more vascular-friendly and flexible double lumen dialysis catheter called Permcath. The tip of the catheter is placed in the superior vena cava close to right atrium and is taken out of the body through a subcutaneous tunnel

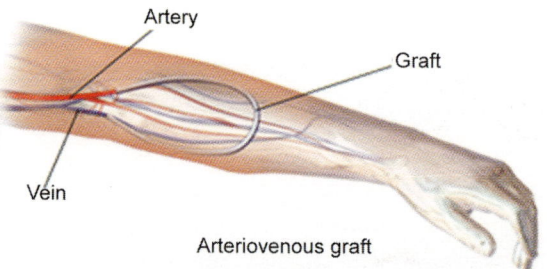

Fig. 24.4: Diagram showing placement of AV graft between brachial artery and cephalic vein at the elbow with PTFE AV graft through the subcutaneous tissue in the forearm in the shape of 'U'.

through the front of the chest (Fig. 24.5). The catheter also has 2 lumens and easily permits blood flow of 300–500 ml per minute. If used carefully, it can be maintained without infection or clotting for many years.

Artificial Kidney (The Dialyser)

There are 2 compartments in the artificial kidney. One compartment is for the blood flow and the other is for dialysate flow. A semi- permeable membrane separates the 2 compartments inside the artificial kidney. When blood and dialysis fluid are made to pass through the artificial kidney continuously throughout the time of dialysis, substances can move from one compartment to the other depending on the principles of osmosis, diffusion and ultrafiltration.

The earliest artificial kidney was made of cuprophane membrane mounted between 2 large flat plates. They have to be assembled to create a blood and dialysis compartment for each dialysis. These plates were heavy, measuring about 3 × 1½ feet and had to be mounted on a stand. Now hollow fiber artificial kidney is used.

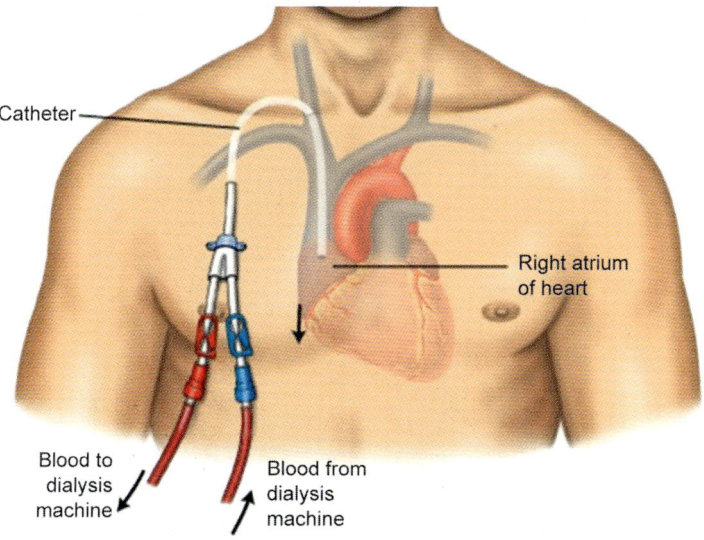

Catheter

Right atrium of heart

Blood to dialysis machine

Blood from dialysis machine

Fig. 24.5: Permanent dialysis catheter (Permcath)—external connections are outside the body. The white part marked catheter goes along subcutaneous tissue in the chest, over the clavicle to the lower neck and bend to enter internal jugular vein. The tip is positioned in junction of superior vena cava and right atrium

The dialysis membrane is manufactured as hollow fibers (thin straw-like tubes). Thousands of such hollow fibers are placed in a housing and sealed at the ends. Thus, 2 separate compartments are formed (Fig. 24.6). The compartment inside the hollow fiber is for blood flow. The space between the fibers is for the flow of dialysis fluid. Thus, the blood and dialysis fluid are separated by the membrane and transport and exchange of substances occur across the membrane. The manufacturer can alter the membrane for different purposes. Artificial kidney with different membranes can be used for different types of dialysis procedures. Membrane can be 'low' or 'high' flux, hemofilter or plasma filter membrane. High flux membrane helps to increase fluid removal and clearance of waste products more efficiently. Hemofilter helps to remove large quantities of ultrafiltrate of plasma in a short time. In hemofiltration, it will be necessary to replace the fluid removed simultaneously. Plasma filter also looks like an artificial kidney. The membrane is

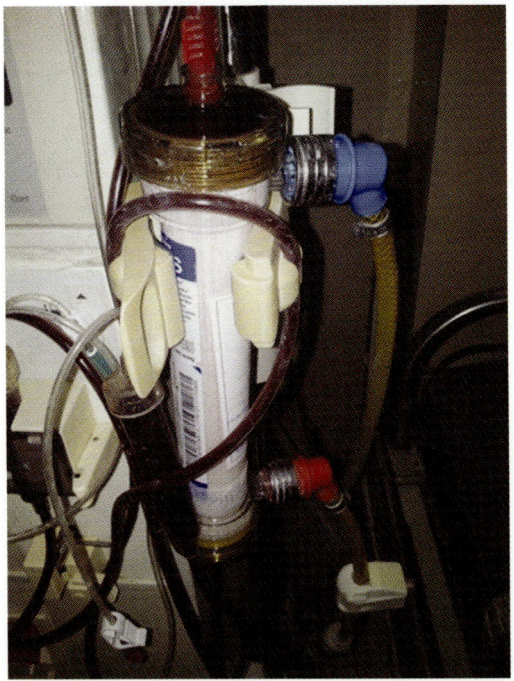

Fig. 24.6: Hollow fiber artificial kidney in use. Bigger blue and red connectors are for dialysis fluid. Smaller red connector for blood line. The small blue connector is in the bottom of the hollow fiber artificial kidney

highly permeable and as the blood flows through, plasma can be removed. Here also plasma and substitutes or fluids should be returned simultanelously, otherwise, the patient may lose a lot of plasma from the body in a short time.

Hemodialysis Monitor (Machine) (Fig. 24.7)

The total quantity of dialysis fluid required for one dialysis is about 120–150 liters. It is not possible to store this quantity by the side of the dialysis bed/couch. So, the fluid needed for dialysis is stored in a concentrated form in suitable cans. The hemodialysis machine prepares the dialysis fluid (dialysate) from the concentrated dialysis fluid in the drum, checks its composition and temperature and circulates it through the artificial kidney. It also circulates the blood from the vascular access through the artificial kidney and back to the patient. There are safety checks on the blood side and dialysate side.

The dialysis machine takes fixed volumes of treated water, hemodialysis concentrates from the drum and appropriate quantity of bicarbonate concentrate from another drum. It mixes the three, heats it to the body temperature, checks the final concentration and temperatue and supplies it to the artificial kidney. If the final

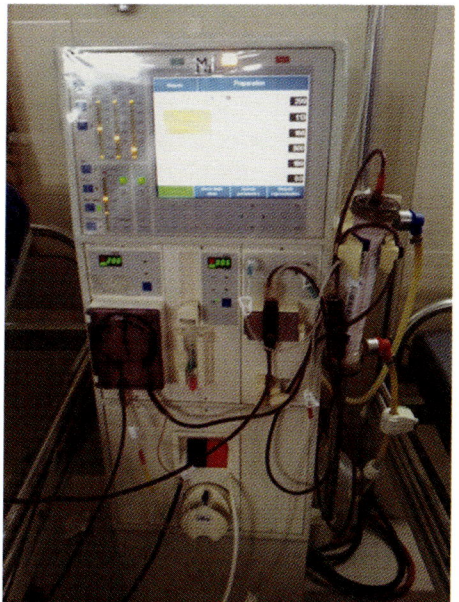

Fig. 24.7: Hemodialysis monitor showing the extracorporeal blood circuit

concentration or temperature is beyond safe limits, it discards the prepared fluid. It also monitors the dialysate circuit and the extracorporeal blood circuit. On the dialysis fluid side, the functions are:

a. Controls flow of dialysate fluid
b. Negative pressure in dialysate compartment (which controls ultrafiltration)
c. Detects blood leak in the artificial kidney
d. Regulates fluid removal from the body
e. Modifies concentration of sodium in the dialysis fluid.
f. Calculates the efficiency of dialysis.

On the blood side, the functions are:
a. Administers heparin at a predetermined rate
b. Pumps to move the blood in the extracorporeal circuit
c. Monitors pressure in the blood tubings
d. Detects air bubbles in the blood and prevents air embolism
e. Monitors blood pressure
f. Gives alarm and stop the dialysis when complications occur
g. Indicates the quantity of fluid removed
h. Indicates the time remaining
i. Self-checks for rinsing, cleaning and disinfection after use.

The dialysis procedure is usually given for 4 hours three times a week when the kidneys fail completely. This will help the patient to lead a near normal life. If strict sterile precautions are not followed, patient may develop infections, septicemia and even die. The water used for dialysis should be treated by filtration, water softener, carbon filter, deionizer and reverse osmosis. Only such purified water should be used. Periodic cultures should be sent from the water source and final purified water. A patient undergoing dialysis is exposed to about 120–150 L of water for every dialysis session. Therefore, the water must be pure and should not contain bacteria or endotoxins.

If kidney failure is temporary, dialysis can be stopped when the kidney function improves further. In case of permanent loss of kidney function, we have to resort to lifelong dialysis or till successful renal transplantation.

Complications which occur during dialysis and their management are summarized in Table 24.1.

In general the complications are divided into acute and chronic complications.

Table 24.1: Complications of hemodialysis and immediate remedies

Acute

Cardiovascular	Hypotension	Most common complication of dialysis. Usually due to excess fluid removal during dialysis. Other causes include poor LV function, autonomic neuropathy, taking food during HD, antihypertensive medications	Rx: Stop ultrafiltration, IV saline bolus, reassess dry weight, Midodrine
	Arrhythmia	Most common arrhythmia is atrial fibrillation. Causes include electrolyte abnormalities, prior cardiovascular disease	Correct electrolyte disturbance, use high potassium dialysate solution
	Hypertension	Removal of antihypertensive medication during dialysis, high calcium concentration of dialysate	Treatment of hypertension
	Sudden cardiac death	Manifestation of ventricular fibrillation/VT or electromechanical dissociation	
Neurological	Dialysis disequilibrium syndrome	Due to osmolal disturbances in the brain leading to cerebral edema	Initiate dialysis slowly, taking care to avoid rapid solute removal, use low blood flow rates and short dialysis time
	Seizures	Could be the manifestation of dialysis disequilibrium syndrome, dialytic removal of antiepileptic drugs or intracranial bleed	Stop dialysis, maintain circulation/airway. Identify cause and treat the cause
Hematological	Hemolysis	Due to altered dialysate composition, raised temperature of dialysate	Stop dialysis and identify cause
Pulmonology	Hypoxemia	Due to RBC sequestration in lungs secondary to complement activation	Rule out dialyzer reactions
Technical	Air embolism, hyponatremia, hypernatremia, Hard water syndrome	Faulty air detector, air enters the blood of hypotension and dyspnea or stroke the patient. Manifests as cardiac arrest	Stop dialysis. place the patient in aspirate air from right ventricle supine position with head end down

CHRONIC COMPLICATIONS

1. Malnutrition
2. Under dialysis
3. Failure of vascular access
4. Bone and mineral disorders—low turnover/high turnover bone disease
5. Dialysis related amyloidosis
6. Acquired cystic renal disease
7. Increased risk of chronic hepatitis B/C infection

Other Modalities of Dialysis

Continuous Renal Replacement Therapy (CRRT)

CRRT is a method of solute and fluid removal in patients with low blood pressure and unstable cardiovascular system. The basic principle is a slow solute and fluid removal. The dialysate flow (about 25–30 ml/min) and blood flow rate (100 ml/min) are kept low. This results in slow solute and fluid removal, maintains plasma osmolality and helps in maintaining hemodynamic stability.

There are many varieties of CRRT

1. Continuous arteriovenous hemofiltration (CAVHF) : Principle of convection
2. Continuous venovenous hemofiltration (CVVHF) : Principle of convection
3. Continuous arteriovenous hemodialysis (CAVHD) : Principle of diffusion
4. Continuous venovenous hemodialysis (CVVHD) : Principle of diffusion
5. Continuous venovenous hemodiafiltration (CVVHDF) : Principle of diffusion and convection (CVVHF and CVVHDF require the use of replacement fluid)

Slow Continuous Ultrafiltration (SCUF)

In this procedure, only ultrafiltration is done at a slow rate. This is particularly useful for removal of body fluids in patients with significant fluid overload but with minimal renal dysfunction, e.g. patients with refractory heart failure.

Hemofiltration

Hemofiltration is a blood purification process using the principle of convection/solvent drag. In this procedure, a highly water permeable membrane called the hemofilter is used. The membrane being extremely permeable to water, removes large quantities of water. Along with the movement of water, solute molecules are also removed by the principle of solvent drag. Dialysis solution is not needed for this procedure. Since large quantity of water is removed during this procedure, a replacement solution which is almost identical in volume and composition to electrolytes in blood is used to replenish the excess fluid loss.

Plasmapheresis

This is an extracorporeal procedure in which the plasma is removed from the blood and replaced with normal fresh frozen plasma. Thus, the plasma from patients which contain disease causing substances or immunoglobulins is separated from the patient's blood, e.g. in Goodpasture's syndrome, antiglomerular basement membrane antibody in plasma is responsible. It causes damage to the glomerular and pulmonary alveolar basement membranes. This procedure is done using a special membrane called plasma filter. When blood passes through the plasma filter, the plasma is filtered and fresh plasma or plasma substitutes are infused with the blood returning to the body. One plasma volume exchange means the removal of the total plasma volume of the patient (about 35–40 ml/kg). The main indications of plasmapheresis include anti-GBM antibody disease, thrombotic thrombocytopenic purpura, Guillain-Barré syndrome and myasthenic crisis.

25

Renal Transplantation

R Kasi Visweswaran, Manu G Krishnan

Renal transplantation is considered when the kidney function is permanently lost and some form of renal replacement therapy is necessary. Lifelong dialysis or renal transplantation is the options before the patient. In maintenance hemodialysis, the patient has to depend on the machine and undergoes dialysis for at least four hours each, three times a week. In CAPD, the procedure is done 3–4 times everyday but the patient is free between the exchanges. After successful renal transplantation, the transplant recipient will have normal kidney function and can resume his regular activity. He will be on lifelong immunosuppressive drug treatment and periodic follow up. Thus, the quality of life after a successful transplantation is superior to other forms of renal replacement therapy.

The person donating the kidney is called the donor and the patient who receives the kidney is called the recipient. In renal transplantation one kidney from a donor is transplanted into the iliac fossa of the recipient. Kidney transplantation is classified based on the source of the donor as living-donor transplantation or deceased-donor (formerly known as cadaveric). Living-donor renal transplants are further characterized as genetically related (living-related) or non-related (living-unrelated) transplants, depending on whether a biological relationship exists between the donor and recipient.

In order to prevent commercial sale of kidneys from donors, the Indian Parliament has enacted the Human Organ Transplantation Act in 1994 and have amended the same from time to time. According to the revised Act, immediate blood relatives are parents, grandparents, brothers, sisters, children, grandchildren and husband or wife. Although husband and wife are not blood relatives, it is legally possible for a husband to donate a kidney to his wife and vice versa. In all these cases, the relationship should be proved legally. In cases of friends, distant relatives or altruistic donors, the request must be considered and cleared by the 'authorising committee' appointed by the Government in every state or region. An informed consent must be obtained from the donor and recipient in the presence of next of kin and witnessed.

DONOR

The donor can be living donor or deceased donor. A living donor is a healthy individual between the ages of 20–60 who has no significant systemic or renal disease and has matching ABO blood group with the recipient. The donor must be aware of the implications of his decision, be willing to donate the kidney and be capable of giving informed consent. If these preliminary conditions are satisfied, he has to undergo physical examination to rule out common systemic diseases like diabetes, severe hypertension, cardiac, pulmonary, renal, psychiatric or neurologic disorders. Investigations like urine routine, 24-hour urine albumin, protein, hemogram and renal function tests are done to rule out renal disease. Subsequently all necessary biochemical tests are done to rule out liver, metabolic or other diseases. Next investigations, ultrasonography and intravenous urography, are done to prove that the donor has 2 kidneys, both are functioning and removal of one will not affect the donor in anyway. Thereafter, investigations like angiography (digital subtraction angiogram {DSA}, CT angiogram or MR angiogram) are done to see the blood supply and the number of blood vessels in each kidney. Human leucocyte antigen (HLA) matching is done to assess the tissue matching between the donor and recipient. Between parent and children, there will be 50% HLA matching. Between siblings, the HLA matching will vary from 0%, 50% or 100%. There is a 25% chance of 0% match, 50% chance of 50% match and 25% chance of 100% matching. Crossmatching between the lymphocytes of the donor and plasma of the recipient is necessary for detecting whether there are antibodies in the recipient against the donor. If the antibodies are present, the kidney will be rejected immediately after transplantation. So such a donor should be rejected. The crossmatch test is repeated on the day prior to transplantation because antibodies may develop at any time. Another source of kidney for live donor transplantation is exchange or swap system. In exchange donation, if the willing donor for a patient A is not matching with patient A but matching with another patient B and the donor of patient B does not match with patient B but matches with patient A, exchange of donors may be considered. The permission of the authorizing committee will be required for the exchange donation.

Deceased donor was formerly called cadaver donor. The process or removing the organs for transplantation is called organ retrieval or organ harvesting. A deceased donor is one who has irreversible brain injury or damage, the brain stem functions are totally lost, who is totally unconscious, has no movements, or spontaneous breathing and who has been supported on artificial means. If such a person, has been certified brain dead independently by 2 teams of doctors at different times, the person can be considered as deceased donor. If the relatives are willing and give informed consent, the person can be taken up as a deceased donor for organ donation. In such an individual, the heart should be beating till the organs are removed. After completing the legal formalities, the following organs can be removed under sterile conditions. The organs are distributed according to the priority list to suitable institutions. Presently, kidneys, liver and occasionally heart are used for transplantation. The following organs can be used for transplantation if facilities are present.

a. Two kidneys
b. Liver
c. Heart
d. Two lungs
e. Pancreas
f. Intestine
g. Two eyes (the eyes can be removed even a few hours after the heart has stopped completely).

RECIPIENT

Noncompliant patients who are not likely to take lifelong medical treatment, those who have incurable malignancy, ongoing substance abuse, morbid obesity, terminal infectious diseases, invalid bedridden patients due to neurological causes and those with no suitable blood vessels for anastamosis are not taken up for transplantation. The recipient should also be prepared prior to transplantation. The recipient should be ambulant, well dialysed, should have hemoglobin >10–11 gm%, should be negative for hepatitis B, C, HIV, tuberculosis, urinary tract infection or any active infection in any part of the body. His cardiac status must be normal and if coronary artery disease is present, he should undergo angioplasty or bypass grafting before transplantation. The recipient must have a gastrointestinal endoscopy to rule out gastric or duodenal ulcer since he will have to take lifelong oral medications. Patients who have 100% chances of recurrence of the original disease in the transplanted kidney are also not considered suitable for receiving the kidney. The iliac blood vessels and the lower urinary tract should also be assessed and found to be suitable before taking up for transplantation.

INDICATIONS FOR RENAL TRANSPLANTATION

End-stage renal disease (ESRD) is the indication for transplantation. ESRD is defined as a glomerular filtration rate <15 ml/min/1.73 sq m. Common diseases leading to ESRD include diabetes mellitus, glomerular diseases, polycystic kidney disease, malignant hypertension, infections, some inborn errors of metabolism and autoimmune diseases with ESRD such as SLE with lupus nephritis. Diabetes is the most common cause of kidney transplantation all over the world. The majority of renal transplant recipients is already on some form of dialysis at the time of transplantation. However, individuals with chronic renal failure who have a living donor available may plan early and undergo transplantation before dialysis is needed. This is called pre-emptive transplantation and is generally advocated in children.

For the recipient, the cultures from blood, urine, sputum are performed about a week prior to the date of transplant. The recipient should be on adequate dialysis and hemoglobin must be maintained without blood transfusions as far as possible. If transfusion is inevitable, WBC free, packed red cells are given through WBC filter and the patient must be on immunosuppressive drugs from 1 day prior to transfusion. A crossmatch test with donor lymphocytes and patients plasma is done 24 hours before surgery to confirm absence of significant antidonor antibodies. The patient is admitted and immunosuppressive drugs started one or two days prior to transplantation as per the protocol of the unit. The recipient is given first dose of basiliximab (simulect—special type of monoclonal antibody against receptor for interleukin-2) 20 mg about an hour before surgery and repeated 72–96 hours after surgery.

TRANSPLANTATION PROCEDURE IN LIVING DONOR TRANSPLANTATION

The donor is prepared with the usual precautions as for a major surgery. The donor is hydrated well so as to achieve a good urine output. The donor undergoes nephrectomy either open or laparoscopic. Simultaneously, the recipient is operated to prepare the bed for the new kidney and expose the iliac artery, vein and dome of the urinary bladder for anastomosis. When the recipient side and perfusion sets are ready, the renal artery, vein and ureter are cut between clamps and the kidney shifted immediately to the perfusion table. It is placed in a basin filled with iced saline flakes, the renal artery canulared and flushed with ice cold solution (Collin's solution or UW solution or Ringer lactate with Heparin and papavarine). This solution will flush out all the blood and cool the core of the kidney. Thus all the blood from the kidney will be washed off and the core and surface of the kidney cooled. The kidney will now look pale and blanched. The time between clamping of the renal artery in the donor and full blanching is called 'warm ischemia' time. It is important to keep this time to the minimum because damage to the kidney may occur if this time is prolonged. The warm ischemia time is variable and is usually 60–150 minutes.

The kidney is now placed in the bed created in the recipient's iliac fossa and covered in iced saline flakes to keep it cool. If the left kidney is removed, it is transplanted in the right iliac fossa and *vice versa*. The renal artery of the donor is anastomosed with the external iliac artery of the recipient (end to side) or internal iliac artery (end to end). The renal vein is anastomosed with the external iliac vein end to side. The recipient is given a dose of methylprednisolone (immunosuppressant medication) before the release of clamps. Once the anastamosis is complete, the ice packs are removed and the clamps released. The time between end of warm ischemia and release of clamps is called 'cold ischemia' time. In live donor transplantation, the cold ischemia time will be equal to the time taken for anastomosis. When the blood from the recipient perfuses the transplanted kidney, the pale and blanched kidney will become pink and usually start producing urine which will come out of the cut end of the ureter. The ureter is now anastomosed to the bladder (Fig. 25.1) and wound closed after placing necessary drains. In the case of deceased donor transplantation, the cold ischemia time may be 24 hours or more since the kidney has to be transported to the center where suitable donors are ready.

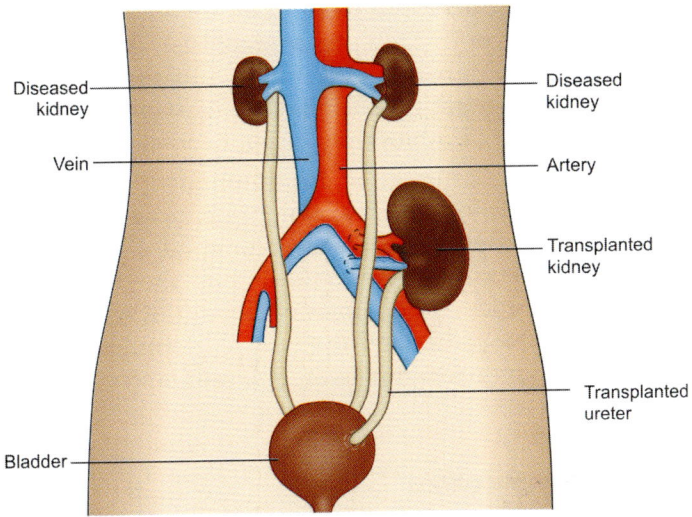

Diseased kidney

Vein

Diseased kidney

Artery

Transplanted kidney

Transplanted ureter

Bladder

Fig. 25.1: Transplanted kidney in left iliac fossa

Note: Renal artery of donor kidney anastomosed to external iliac artery—end to side, renal vein to external iliac vein—end to side and ureter to bladder. The old diseased kidneys and ureters remain after transplantation.

Postoperatively, the donor requires the routine care as for a nephrectomy in a postoperative ward and discharged in 5–7 days. The donor may avoid heavy manual work and be on rest for a few weeks as for a major surgery. Annual checkup is advised thereafter.

The recipient is closely monitored in an independent ICU with 'Barrier nursing'. The fluid intake output, blood pressure, CVP, drain volume, temperature and pulse, are monitored hourly. The fluid intake adjusted every half to 1 hour depending on the output volume. Many recipients may have very high urine output even more than 10–12 liters in 24 hours for a few days. The hemoglobin, hematocrit, blood counts, blood sugar, renal functions and serum electrolytes including bicarbonate are monitored at least twice a day initially. Immunosuppressive medications are continued by parenteral route on the first day and later changed to oral. The hourly fluid intake is regulated by the blood pressure, CVP and fluid output. After successful transplantation, the renal function test becomes normal in about 72 hours. A second dose of simulect is given between 48 and 72 hours post-transplant.

The immunosuppressive drugs can be induction agents (corticosteroids, ATG or IL-2 receptor antagonists). The maintenance drugs are corticosteroids, calcinurin inhibitors (CNIs → cyclosporine/tacrolimus), mTOR inhibitors (sirolimus, everolimus) and antimetabolites (azathioprine, mycophenolate).

Earlier, the three drugs used for immunosuppression were, prednisolone, cyclosporine and azathioprine. Now, prednisolone, tacrolimus and mycophenolate are used commonly. The blood level of tacrolimus is monitored periodically and the dose adjusted. Other drugs like intravenous immunoglobulin (IVIg), sirolimus, everolimus, azathioprine, anti-thymocyte globulin (ATG), and interleukin-2 receptor antagonists are also used in specific situations.

COMPLICATIONS

Immediate Complications

a. *Hyperacute rejection:* Due to antibodies in the recipient against the donor cells. This results in immediate graft loss and the transplanted kidney will not function and has to be removed immediately. It is rare and pre-transplant crossmatch test will help to identify such patients. If pre-transplant crossmatch is positive, the surgery is not undertaken. The surgery is under-taken only after crossmatch becomes negative.

b. *Surgical complications:* Bleeding, thrombosis at the site of anastomosis, urinary leak.

c. *Acute rejection:* May occur during the early weeks or up to first 6 months. Patient may develop fever, graft swelling, oliguria, elevation of creatinine or increased leucocyte excretion in urine. Treatment is by antirejection protocols, mainly increasing the dose of immunosuppressive drugs. There are two types of acute rejection—acute cellular rejection and acute vascular rejection.

d. *Hypertension:* May worsen after transplantation due to drugs used as immunosuppression or due to stenosis of the trans-planted renal artery. If the graft is functioning well, the hyper-tension may subside.

e. *Primary graft dysfunction:* In this condition, there is no improvement of renal function after transplantation and the patient needs dialysis to maintain the kidney function. This may be due to many causes. If it is due to prolonged ischemia periods, both warm and cold, the tubules may be damaged and recovery is possible after a few days or weeks.

f. *Infections:* Since the immune system of the patient is suppressed, any type of infection could occur after transplantation. There can be flare up of hidden infections or new bacterial, viral, protozoal, rickettsial or fungal infections.

g. *Post-transplant diabetes mellitus (PTDM):* Development of diabetes mellitus in a nondiabetic recipient after renal transplantation is call PTDM. The drugs used for immunosuppression like tacrolimus and prednisolone are often responsible.

h. Post-transplant malignancies: Lymphoproliferative diseases (PTLD) occur many years after transplantation. Hodgkin's lymphoma, and other malignancies occur more in transplanted individuals compared to general population.

i. Post-transplant dyslipidemia, bone disease and recurrence of the disease in the transplanted kidneys are the other complications.

j. After many years of transplantation, the kidney function may worsen gradually when there is chronic rejection.

It is necessary to monitor each transplant recipient periodically for these complications so that early diagnosis can be made and therapy started.

The number of persons with kidney disease needs renal transplantation is increasing. Because of the nuclear family system, the number of related donors is less. Restriction on organ trade and illegal transplantations have made procedure more elaborate for nonrelated living donor transplantation. It is possible to use organs from a deceased donor (earlier known as cadaver donor) for transplantation. Organs like kidneys, liver, heart, lungs, intestine have to be removed from a brain dead person after completing all legal formalities before cardiac arrest or clinical death occurs. Once cardiac arrest occurs and circulation stops, these organs become unfit for transplantation. Only the cornea can be taken within hours from a clinically dead person. Under these circumstances, enlarging the pool of deceased donors by health education and counseling should be encouraged.

26

Diet in Kidney Diseases

Jose Paul, R Kasi Visweswaran

Although we consume various types of diet, the volume and composition of the body is maintained within a normal range. The kidneys play a very important role in regulating water and electrolyte balance. It also helps to excrete the waste products and prevent accumulation of waste in the body. In a patient with kidney disease, the diet should be suitably modified so that accumulation of waste products in the body is minimized. Our diet contains carbohydrates, proteins, fats, water, minerals, fibres and vitamins. The daily diet should provide energy for daily activities and growth.

Normal individuals need about 30–40 kcal/kg body weight/day of energy approximately as carbohydrates 70%, fats 20% and proteins 10% respectively. Carbohydrates provide 4 kcal energy/gm and fat provides 9 kcal energy/gm. These are broken down to CO_2 and H_2O and liberate ATP (adenosine triphosphate) which is the source of energy. The proteins also provide 4 kcal/gm of energy. They are broken down to urea, sulfuric acid and phosphoric acid. The nuclei in the cells contain nucleic acid and its metabolism yields uric acid. The carbon dioxide is eliminated through expired air. These acids together with urea, creatinine, uric acid and water have to be excreted by the kidneys.

It will be necessary to estimate the ideal body weight to calculate the calorie requirement for a patient. The actual body weight may be more in edematous conditions and low in malnourished patients. An approximate ideal body weight can be calculated by the following:

Ideal body weight (kg) = Height in cm – 100
Example: The ideal body weight in a patient with height of 160 cm will be 160 – 100 = 60 kg.

It is necessary to understand two concepts before prescribing diet for patients, namely diet plan and meal plan. Diet plan is decided based on weight and age of the patient, nature of kidney disease, associated abnormalities, presence of edema, level of kidney functions, volume of output, level of consciousness, drugs to be used and other factors. Based on this, the physician prescribes the diet plan. The diet plan for 20-year male weighing 60 kg who has acute kidney injury due to crush injury (road traffic accident) has urine output of 300 ml in 24 hours and worsening renal function is given in the example.

Example: Diet plan

Energy	–	2100 kcal (35 kcal/kg)
Protein	–	1.6 gm (0.6 gm/kg)
Distribution of carbohydrates and fats	–	4 : 1
Fluids	–	800 ml (output volume + 500 ml)
Salt	–	2 gm
Potassium	–	No potassium

Semi-liquid diet

The dietician provides a palatable oral diet or Ryle's tube feed by providing the actual ingredients according to the prescribed diet plan. This is called meal plan.

Example: Meal plan. (No fruits or fruit juices/volume of fluids not to exceed 800 ml.)

6 am	–	Milk (150 ml) with sugar 1tbsp
8 am	–	Breakfast as porridge
11 am	–	Low potassium food
1 pm	–	Lunch—semi-liquid with vegetables, powdered rice-porridge, egg white/fish
4 pm	–	Milk and salt-free biscuits
7 pm	–	Supper
10 pm	–	Bedtime snacks

For **acute kidney injury**, if the patient has oliguria, the diet should include "fluid restriction, salt restriction, potassium free diet with protein 0.6 gm/kg (at least) and calories 35 kcal/kg. The diet may be modified based on clinical condition whether dialysis is given, urine output volume or presence of fever.

Diet in **chronic renal failure** should also contain a minimum of 0.6 gm protein/kg. In India the protein intake of an average non-vegetarian is <1.2 gm/kg and in the case of vegetarian <0.5 gm/kg. Protein restriction is advised only for those taking protein intake of >1.5 gm/kg. For most of our patients, advise to restrict to fish and egg white is recommended everyday and lean meat (chicken) once in a week will provide an average of 0.6 gm/kg protein, vegetarians need not restrict pulses and cereals as quantity consumed is not excessive and will seldom exceed 0.6 gm/kg. The calorie requirement is about 30 kcal/kg/day. Sodium restriction is advised if the patient has hypertension or edema. Otherwise, only high salt food needs to be avoided.

Diet in **nephritic syndrome** should be fluid and salt restriction. The protein intake should be normal approximately 0.8 to 1.0 gm/kg in adult and 1.5 to 1.8 gm/kg in children.

In **renal stone disease**, fluid intake is generally increased so that the urine is dilute. The chances of formation or growth of stones is less if the urine is dilute. Moreover, if there is constant formation and flow of urine through the urinary system, small stones may be carried down to the bladder and excreted. Green leafy vegetables contain oxalate may be avoided if urinary oxalate is high. If uric acid is high, red meat, dry fish, etc have to be avoided.

Patients **who are on dialysis** may consume normal food avoiding excessive fluid intake and potassium rich diet (fruits, fruit juices, soft drinks). They are monitored regularly and must be advised to restrict weight gain between 2 dialysis sessions to <2.5 kg.

Foods to be avoided/limited in patients on maintenance hemodialysis. Nuts and berries, citrus fruits, banana, soft drinks, food high in salt content, e.g. canned meat/fish.

Those on **CAPD (continuous ambulatory peritoneal dialysis)** lose protein in the peritoneal fluid drained after dialysis and since they lose a lot of protein, they are advised very high protein diet— even 3–4 gm protein/kg to compensate for the losses. The fluid intake and daily weight are checked to decide on the permitted volume of fluid intake.

In CKD patients on dialysis with severe malnutrition and not responding to oral dietary interventions, total parenteral nutrition in the form of **intra-dialytic parenteral nutrition (IDPN)** may be attempted.

Thus, diet plays an important part of treatment of renal diseases and a good diet plan and palatable meal plan will help the patient to comply with the restrictions necessary for successful treatment.

27

Psychiatric Aspects of Renal Diseases

Jose Paul

Diagnosis of kidney disease in a member of the family is a shocking experience for the whole family. There is great stress on the patient and family members. Since most of the major treatment methods are very expensive it adds to further stress.

The psychiatric aspects of kidney disease may be broadly classified as:

1. Due to renal failure
2. Due to involvement of other systems
3. Due to prolonged and expensive treatment
4. Due to restriction on diet and activity
5. Interpersonal relationship with members of family and staff in treatment unit.

Renal disease may be associated with delirium, dementia or amnesia. Patients with renal disease may have anxiety, alterations in mood, fatigue, depression, sexual dysfunction, irritability and insomnia. All these may affect the mental health of the patient. Some may develop behavioral symptoms or even frank psychiatric illness. The family members and caregivers of the patient with chronic illness of the kidney are also under great stress. Attending the patients on regular dialysis or renal transplant recipients is stressful for staff in the renal unit. Proper approach, counseling and use of drugs when needed will help to keep these patients more comfortable.

Depression is very common and leads to increased psychological stress and mortality. It is an important factor and determines the long-term prognosis. Those with depressive illness at the onset of dialysis do poorly in the long-term. Low levels of social support, compliance and lack of awareness contribute to increased mortality.

Suicide is more common in dialysis patients. Severe financial constraints, lack of social support and alcohol/drug dependence are important associated factors. Under dialysis, cerebrovascular disease and drug and alcohol dependence and uremic encephalopathy are other organic factors which may contribute to depression. Psychological and social support is a crucial component of the treatment plan. Antidepressants are effective in 75% of patients. They take about 4–6 weeks for full effect. Since most of the antidepressants are metabolized in the liver, dosage modification is not generally required.

The renal conditions which cause psychiatric illness are related to uremia, hyponatremia, hypocalcemia, hypercalcemia, hyperphosphatemia and metabolic acidosis. Complications of renal failure like anemia, hypertension, hypertensive encephalopathy, cardiac failure, endocrine disorders, sepsis and stroke can affect the mental status. The role of medications dialysis, interpersonal factors in renal transplantation are also responsible for the psychological changes.

Dementia and delirium are more common in elderly dialysis patients. Dementia occurs early in those with metabolic abnormalities of uremia. Other causes include Alzheimer's disease and various forms of dementia. Aluminium related dementia is now uncommon in dialysis patients due to better water quality and the avoidance of aluminium containing phosphate binders. Dialysis patients have an increased risk of stroke and vascular dementia than in the general population.

Dialysis disequilibrium is a condition due to rapid removal of urea from the blood stream at the time of starting dialysis treatment. When the level of urea decrease suddenly, the urea from the cells in the brain do not diffuse rapidly. Higher osmolarity of the intracellular compartment results in edema of the brain and symptoms of dementia. This is called dialysis disequilibrium syndrome.

Water-soluble vitamins are dialysed and removed from the body. Such patients should get replacement with vitamins B and C. Thiamine deficiency can result in acute neurological complications.

'Bystander burn out': The need for constant care and sometimes, noncooperative attitude of the patient towards treatment and caregivers may lead to frustration and depression in the caregiver at home.

The staff working with non-cooperative chronic patients are also under great stress.

28

Comprehensive Nursing in Nephrology

SR Terese Kochuvilayil, R Kasi Visweswaran

It is important to look into three aspects of nursing when looking after a patient with renal disease.

1. Nursing and diagnostic tests
2. Nursing management in renal diseases
3. Nursing management in renal replacement therapies

NURSING IN DIAGNOSTIC TESTS

One of the important duties of the nurse is to collect, label and send the samples correctly to the laboratory. The method of collection, and transport to the laboratory has a great role in getting accurate and reliable reports in time. All samples must be collected properly in the appropriate container. The sample should be labelled correctly with name of patient, age, gender, room/ward, identification number, name of doctor who ordered the test, diagnosis, and the tests requested. The request slip should be signed with name and designation of the person signing the request. The name of the requesting doctor in the requisition slip is important because the laboratory can contact the doctor immediately when there is a serious abnormality in the test which has to be brought to the notice urgently. In all cases, precautions are taken to protect the caregiver. The 'universal precautions' should be followed while handling blood and body fluids in all patients irrespective of whether they have infection or not. The label "BBF" (blood and body fluids) should be attached to the request form and the sample bottle if the sample is from HbsAg, HCV or HIV positive patients according to the respective hospital's protocol.

The main principles in urine collection are to give correct instructions to the patient for collecting urine samples. Example: To collect the whole voided first sample in the morning/midstream sample/collecting 3 samples in 3 glasses at the beginning, middle and end of micturition/24-hour urine/urine for culture and sensitivity. The external genitalia should be cleaned with water, foreskin retracted (in males) or labia separated (in females). There should be no contamination from foreskin or vulva. In women, preferably urine sample should not be taken during periods. If it is taken during periods, it must be mentioned. Urine sample should be despatched to the laboratory immediately, otherwise decomposition may occur. If any delay is anticipated, appropriate preservative is added to the urine. The important precaution for collecting 24-hour or timed urine collections is that the patient should empty the bladder at the time of starting collection. This is not to be collected since it represents the urine which has been formed before the collection period.

Prenursing for radiographic procedures (plain X-ray, CT scan, intravenous urogram, micturating cystourethrogram, contrast CT urogram and other types of pyelograms) include use of laxative, cathartics or enema previous day evening, advice light supper and nil orally from midnight, check iodine or shellfish allergies and send the patient for the procedure in the morning. This will help best visualisation of kidneys in radiologic studies. If the X-ray is delayed, gas may accumulate in the abdomen following involuntary swallowing of air. Informed written consent is taken as per the hospital protocol and the patient is explained about the procedure. Postprocedure nursing involves observing the urine output, looking for hematuria allergies to dye or sepsis.

Renal angiography, aortography, selective angiography are studies where a catheter is introduced through femoral artery and contrast medium is injected. The passage of the dye through the renal artery, renal capillaries, venous system, and excretion through ureter and bladder. Serial X-rays or videography are used to study the same. In addition to the regular prenursing care for radiologic studies, blood tests for renal function are necessary because the radiocontrast media can worsen renal function. Appropriate additional measures will be necessary if the kidney function is deranged. The special precautions in postnursing care are applying pressure bandage over injection sites in the artery, bed rest 12 to 24 hours, checking the site for hematoma formation, monitoring vital signs including peripheral pulse distal to the site. The urine output must be monitored since oliguria or polyuria may occur.

Renal biopsy is an invasive investigation. The needle of the biopsy gun is introduced up to the renal cortex under local anesthesia and a sample of kidney is obtained to determine the histology of glomeruli and tubules. For renal biopsy, the special requirements are to check coagulation studies and hematocrit. After the biopsy, pressure dressing is applied over insertion site and patient is placed in prone position for 30 to 60 minutes and maintain bed rest for 24 hours. The vital signs are monitored, patient is given adequate fluids and regular diet. Urine samples are collected to look for gross hematuria. The patient should be assessed for flank pain, hypotension, decreased hematocrit, temperature elevation, chills, urinary frequency and dysuria. The patient is permitted to move about after 24 hours.

NURSING MANAGEMENT IN COMMON RENAL DISEASES

The individual renal diseases are more fully described in the respective chapters. Only the nursing assessment and management of some common kidney diseases are highlighted in this chapter.

Acute Glomerulonephritis

Patients with acute glomerulonephritis often present with sudden onset of facial puffiness, oliguria, hypertension, headache, shortness of breath due to fluid retention, weakness, visual problems or flank pain. Objective assessment may show hematuria, proteinuria, puffiness and edema legs, hypertension, oliguria, proteinuria, urinary casts, elevated urea, creatinine. If the glomerulonephritis is due to previous streptococcal infection, elevated antistreptolysin O (ASO) titer may be observed. Most patients recover. Some may develop complications.

Nursing Interventions

a. Monitor vital signs
b. Fluid I/O to be charted accurately
c. Daily weight chart and check for subsidence of edema and look for pulmonary edema
d. Provide bed rest until clinical symptoms resolve
e. Explain diagnostic test, condition, and treatment and provide emotional support
f. Monitor blood urea, serum creatinine and urinalysis.

g. Sodium and fluid restriction based on urine output/edema/ weight

h. Diuretics, antihypertensives and antibiotics as prescribed

i. Diet which is low in sodium and protein but high in carbohydrate and calories

j. Protect against infection or injury

k. Explain home care and maintenance and follow up.

Even though the symptoms subside, these patients should be on periodic and long-term follow up.

Nephrotic Syndrome

Nephrotic syndrome is a common renal disease associated with loss of large quantities of protein in the urine. As a result, hypoalbuminemia develops. This leads to edema, hyperlipidemia and sometimes even hypertension and renal failure. The subject is discussed separately in an earlier chapter.

Nursing Interventions

a. Assessment and care for severely edematous patient

b. Monitoring vital signs

c. Monitoring daily weight (severely edematous patients should lose 0.5 to 1.0 kg weight everyday if the fluid intake is regulated correctly.)

d. Accurate fluid intake output chart and nursing care to control edema

e. Regulated salt and fluid intake

f. Periodic urine and blood examination

g. Diet with low salt, low fluids, low fat and normal protein (such patients often have loss of appetite)

h. Psychological support

i. Administer drugs as prescribed (corticosteroids, diuretics, antihypertensive drugs, antacids, vitamins)

j. Adequate rest and assess for signs of infection (immune system is often depressed)

k. Administer salt—poor albumin to reduce fluid retention (Albumin infusions help to reduce edema and increase the efficiency of diuretics.)

l. Observe for pulmonary edema: Tachypnea, dyspnea

m. Use good handwashing and infection control techniques

n. Avoid or minimize invasive procedures

Urinary Tract Infections

Urinary tract infection means invasion of urinary tract by pathogenic bacteria. The infection can be in the lower urinary tract alone or mainly in upper urinary tract. Upper urinary tract includes the kidneys, renal pelvis and ureters. Pyelonephritis is infection of upper urinary tract. Clinical manifestations are fever, chills, malaise, flank pain, costovertebral tenderness, tachypnea, urinary frequency and dysuria. Constitutional symptoms like fever chills, GI symptoms, muscle tenderness are more common in pyelonephritis. In lower tract infection, symptoms like painful micturition, severe burning sensation, painful sensation of incomplete bladder emptying and frequency of micturition are more common.

Nursing Interventions

a. Sending for urine routine and culture before starting treatment (pyuria, bacteriuria leukocyte casts hematuria)
b. Blood examination (leukocytosis, rule out diabetes, renal function tests if ordered)
c. Maintain bed rest until symptoms subside
d. Encourage large fluid intake to maintain urine output of 1500 ml/day.
e. Monitor urine for presence of pus cells, RBCs, bacteria
f. Monitor blood counts and RFT
g. Control diabetes if diabetic
h. Observe for edema and signs of renal failure
i. Antibiotic course to be completed, urinary antiseptics, and analgesics for pain.

Polycystic Kidney Disease

Polycystic kidney disease is an inherited disorder and the correct name is autosomal dominant polycystic kidney disease (ADPKD). It is common and may be present in many members of the same family. The manifestations start only after middle ages. The patient may be asymptomatic, have hypertension, Flank or abdominal pain, fever and chills due to UTI or infection of cyst, malaise, hematuria, hypertension, palpable abdominal masses due to enlarged kidneys.

Nursing Interventions

a. Monitor vital signs, and intake output chart (if hospitalised)
b. Collect urine for culture

c. Monitor for gross hematuria, or signs of cyst rupture

d. Avoid urinary catheters to prevent infection

e. Administer antibiotics and analgesics as prescribed

f. Instruct bed rest in case of ruptured cysts and bleeding

g. Provide psychological support

h. Explain procedures, condition and management

i. Explain home care/signs of infection/medications/treatment plan

j. Family counselling on inherited disease

k. Follow-up care.

Renal Calculi

Urinary stones form from a 'nidus' or a focus within the urinary system. The stone crystals formed when the urine is concentrated accumulate around the nidus and form stones. Stones may form from calcium, cystine, oxalates, phosphates and uric acid. The calcium and cystine stones are visible on plain X-ray (radiopaque). Uric acid stones are not seen in plain X-ray (radiolucent). The stone may remain without any symptom, grow in size and number gradually, cause pain, obstruction, bleeding or kidney damage.

Nursing Interventions

a. Assess severity of symptoms

b. Observe for stone growth (this requires follow-up every 6 months if the stone is 'silent' which does not cause any symptom or causing damage).

c. *Observe for symptoms:* Pain (colic), bleeding (hematuria), obstruction (hydronephrosis), infection (UTI) or renal damage (renal failure).

d. *Confirm presence, position, size and whether causing block (investigations as ordered:* X-ray (KUB), IVP, retrograde pyelography, urinalysis, ultrasound, cystoscopy or MRI).

e. Monitor urine output, note reaction and appearance (some stones form in acidic and some in alkaline urine)

f. Strain all urine (if stone fragments are present preserve for stone analysis)

g. Administer prescribed analgesics and antispasmodics

h. Encourage oral fluid of 2500 ml/day (to facilitate passage of stone and prevent infection)

i. Administer necessary IV fluids as prescribed.

j. Explain diagnostic procedures and treatments

k. Monitor renal functions and electrolytes.

l. Provide appropriate nursing care for treatment chosen.

END Stage Renal Failure (ESRD)

In ESRD, the kidney function is permanently lost and the kidney function assessed by GFR is less than 15 ml/min. This represents stage 5 of chronic kidney disease by the recent classification. Once confirmed, such patients will need 'renal replacement therapy' which may be in the form of lifelong dialysis or renal transplantation. The symptoms can be highly variable and relate to almost any system in the body.

Nursing Interventions Include

a. Monitor fluid I/O, blood pressure, weight charts and laboratory values

b. *Diet:* Protein 0.8 g/kg body weight (low protein diet is not necessary for our patients since most of them are already on low protein diet) and potassium free diet.

c. Regulated fluid depending on output, salt restriction

d. Administer medication as ordered

e. Teach the patient regarding weight, fluid intake, dietary restrictions, avoid nephrotoxic drugs, fruits/fruit juices.

f. Strategies to avoid thirst (frequent mouth care, sugarless hard candy, use ice chips and spray water)

g. Counselling and preparation for renal replacement therapy.

NURSING MANAGEMENT IN RENAL REPLACEMENT THERAPIES

Peritoneal Dialysis

In peritoneal dialysis, hypertonic dialysing solution (dialysate) is instilled under sterile precautions through the catheter into peritoneal cavity. Excess of electrolytes and uremic toxins move by diffusion across peritoneal membrane into dialysis solution. Water removal by osmosis can be modified by increasing the glucose concentration (increase osmolality) of the PD solution. Nursing cares for peritoneal catheter insertion are:

a. Empty bladder and bowel (if necessary urinary catheter and/or enema).

b. Weigh the patient.

c. Written informed consent.

d. Monitor vital signs
e. Skin preparation from nipple line to mid thigh
f. Set up the sterile tray, catheter set and dialysis solutions
g. After the insertion of catheter clean the area with antiseptic solution and sterile dressing is applied
h. Irrigate with heparinised dialysate (to clear blood and fibrin from catheter).
i. Instruct the patient to keep the dressing dry
j. For CAPD it is preferable to allow a waiting period of 7 to 14 days.
k. Once the catheter site is healed, the patient can take shower and pat the area to dry.
l. Daily care and observation for signs of infection at the insertion site.
m. For IPD, the catheter can be used immediately.

The complications are infection, obstruction by clots or fibrin, one-way obstruction to flow of fluid, hypotension (excess fluid removal), abdominal fullness (fluid in peritoneum), hyperglycemia (high glucose concentration in dialysis solution), protein loss in dialysis fluid. Patients on CAPD should be advised high protein diet (2–2.5 g protein/kg/day).

Care of an Arteriovenous (AV) Fistula

AV fistula provides vascular access through a superficial vein for hemodialysis. Since the vein is directly connected with an artery, the blood flow is high. Even during the early stages of renal failure, it is preferable to maintain one arm without venepunctures for future AV fistula. Before surgery, the circulation to the limb and suitability of blood vessels are checked. An artificial internal connection is made between the artery and neighboring vein. A bruit will be heard over the vein. In about 6–8 weeks, the vein will enlarge, the wall of the vein will become thickened and blood flow will increase. This is called maturing of AV fistula. It can be used for hemodialysis only after it has become mature. The working of AV fistula is made by auscultating for bruits and palpating for thrills. Lack of bruit may indicate block or blood clot and requires immediate attention. The arm with fistula should not be used for BP measurements, venepuncture for blood sampling and lifting heavy objects. There should be a dressing after dialysis to prevent bleeding but the tourniquet should not obstruct the blood flow.

Home Care Instructions

a. Keep fistula area clean and dry
b. Notify if pain, swelling, redness or drainage in accessed arm
c. Avoid excessive pressure to arm
d. Do not sleep with the arm supporting the head, wear tight clothing or jewellery.
e. Keep the area dry for 4–6 hours after dialysis.

Hemodialysis

Hemodialysis is done to remove waste products from the blood and maintain fluid and electrolyte balance.

Pre-procedural Nursing Care

a. Weigh the patient, take vital signs, including BP in sitting and standing position
b. Withhold routine medications until dialysis complete
c. Wear protective eyewear, gown and gloves
d. Monitor blood tests at the beginning and end of dialysis according to the hospital protocol
e. Early in course of haemodialysis, look for and report dialysis disequilibrium syndrome. (It is the development of fresh neurologic symptoms like headache, mental confusion, decreased level of consciousness, nausea, vomiting, twitching and even seizure during dialysis. It may be due to cerebral edema when blood urea is removed rapidly. It can be prevented by dialyzing for shorter times or at reduced blood flow rates early in course of therapy.)
f. Monitor for hypotension, clotting time and partial thromboplastin time (to confirm proper dose of anticoagulation)
g. Monitor and correct the alarm situations indicated by the machine promptly.
h. At the end of treatment, return blood remaining in the dialyzer and tube to the patient and remove needles from vascular access.
i. Apply tourniquet with correct pressure at the site of insertion of needle in AV fistula. For catheters, apply cap and give sterile dressing.

Renal Transplantation

Nursing care is very important in a patient who undergoes renal transplantation. The care starts weeks before transplantation and will go on lifelong for the recipient of the transplant.

Preoperative Nursing Care

a. Teach about procedure and reduce anxiety for donor and recipient.
b. Administer immunosuppressive drugs, discuss purpose and possible adverse effects with client, monitor for increased BP and signs of anaphylaxis
c. Plan for client to undergo dialysis the day before surgery
d. Plan for cleaning enema and many laboratory tests.

Postoperative Care

a. Perform baseline assessments: Vital signs, nursing care, status of dressing.
b. Encourage early mobility and breathing exercises
c. Use special aseptic techniques and standard universal precautions to control infection.
d. Observe for signs of tissue rejection: Fever, tenderness and swelling at surgical site, WBC, urine output with proteinuria, sudden weight gain, hypertension, elevated BUN and creatinine
e. Provide analgesics as per order
f. Monitor urine output closely, report output less than 100 ml/hour, decreased urine output may indicate thrombus formation at renal artery anastomosis site.
g. Expect blood tinged urine for several days and irrigate catheter with aseptic technique.

With a living donor transplant, urine flow should begin immediately after revascularization and connection of ureter to client's bladder, with a cadaver transplant, expect anuria for 2 days to 2 weeks; client will need dialysis during this period
- Monitor daily RFT
- Observe for signs of hyperkalemia
- Weigh patient daily

Home Management

a. Measure and record I/O chart, notify if urine output <600 ml/day
b. Instruct how to collect urine, 24-hour urine sample
c. Advice to weigh twice weekly
d. Drink water depending on urine output volume and climatic condition.
e. Avoid smoking and excessive alcohol.
f. Report signs of rejection: Redness, warmth, tenderness or swelling over the kidney, fever, urinary output, BP
g. Avoid crowded places for 3–6 months after surgery
h. Practice regular, moderate exercise regularly.

Fluid, Electrolyte and Acid–Base Balance

29

Body Fluids and IV Fluids

R Kasi Visweswaran

DISTRIBUTION OF WATER IN THE BODY

About 60% of the body weight is water. The percentage of water content will be more in children, lean persons and males compared to older, obese females. This is distributed in the body in different compartments. These compartments are not water tight. There is always movement of fluids between the body fluid compartments. The fluid is distributed either inside the cell or outside the cell. The fluid inside the cell is called intracellular fluid (ICF). The outside the cell is called extracellular and is in 3 different compartments. They are:

a. Interstitial—About 70%: This is called the interstitial or extracellular fluid (ECF).
b. Intravascular—about 25% and
c. Transcellular—about 5%.

Interstitial fluid surrounds the cells and is outside the blood vessels. The intravascular water is within the blood vessels. Transcellular fluids include the cerebrospinal fluid (CSF), fluids within the eyes, joints and lymph (Fig. 29.1).

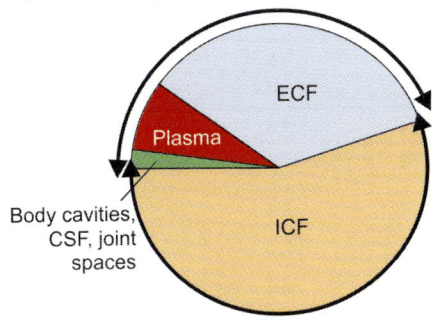

Fig. 29.1: Distribution of body water

By weight, the distribution is as follows:

Total body water   = 60% of body weight (varies from 45 to 75%)

ICF   = 40% of body weight

ECF   = 15% of body weight

Intravascular (blood) = 5% of body weight

The thirst mechanism of the brain controls the water intake. When we drink liquids, it is absorbed by the intestines, carried through the blood to different parts of the body. From the capillaries, the fluid moves into the ECF and to the ICF. Since continuous exchange of fluids occurs between the various compartments, it is said to be in dynamic equilibrium.

COMPOSITION OF FLUIDS IN VARIOUS BODY COMPARTMENTS

It is important to understand the differences in the composition of intracellular and extracellular fluids. Sodium is the most abundant **cation** (see box) in ECF, potassium is the most abundant cation in intracellular fluid. The blood plasma and ECF contain mainly sodium, chloride and bicarbonate. There is more calcium in the blood compared to ECF.

Understanding cations and anions

Cation: It is a positively charged ion which moves to the cathode (negative end) of the electrical circuit, e.g. Na^+, K^+, Ca^{2+}, Mg^{2+}, NH_4^+. Cations have positive charge and are given '+' sign.

Anion: It is a negatively charged ion which moves to the anode (positive end) of the electrical circuit. It is denoted by '−' sign, e.g. Cl^-, HCO_3^-, PO_4^{3-}.

The ICF contains mainly potassium, magnesium and phosphate. The calcium and bicarbonate contents are very low (Table 29.1).

Table 29.1: Electrolyte composition of ICF and ECF			
	Intracellular fluid (mEq / L)	Interstitial fluid (mEq /L)	Plasma (mEq /L)
Sodium	10	140	140 ± 4
Potassium	150	4–5	4.5 ± 1
Chloride	2	104	102 ± 4
Bicarbonate	6	24	24 ± 2
Calcium	0.01	5	10 ± 1 mg %
Magnesium	40	3.0	0.8 – 1.2
Phosphate/sulphate	150	8.0	—

There is a 'pump' called Na$^+$, K$^+$-ATPase pump in the cell wall of all cells. This pump pushes sodium out of the cell and moves potassium inside the cell by using energy. So this is called active transport. Therefore, the ICF compartment is the "home" of potassium (Fig. 29.2). The number of anions and cations in each compartment will be equal. Anions like Cl$^-$ and HCO$_3^-$ and cations like Na$^+$, K$^+$, Ca^{++} and Mg^{++} can be measured in blood.

It is necessary to know the composition of fluids in various body secretions because this will help us to replace the fluid lost due to various disorders correctly. The gastric juice is highly **acidic** (see box below) and contains chloride in the form of hydrochloric acid. Duodenal secretions contain a lot of potassium and some sodium. Pancreatic juice is highly alkaline and is rich in sodium bicarbonate. Bile and jejunal secretions are rich in sodium and chloride, whereas ileal secretions contain more of bicarbonate and less of sodium. It is necessary to know which type of fluid is lost from the GIT to decide about the replacement fluid required.

Understanding acids and alkali (base)

Acid: Acids are substances which can donate hydrogen ions (H$^+$) when in aqueous solution. It has low pH. Acids have a sour taste and **turn blue litmus red.** When an acid is added to a solution, the H$^+$ concentration increases and pH goes down.

Base–alkali: Bases are substances which accept hydrogen ions and yield hydroxide (OH$^-$) ions when in aqueous solution. It increases the pH. Bases have a bitter taste, feel greasy and **turn red litmus blue.** When alkali is added to a solution, the H$^+$ concentration decreases and pH goes up.

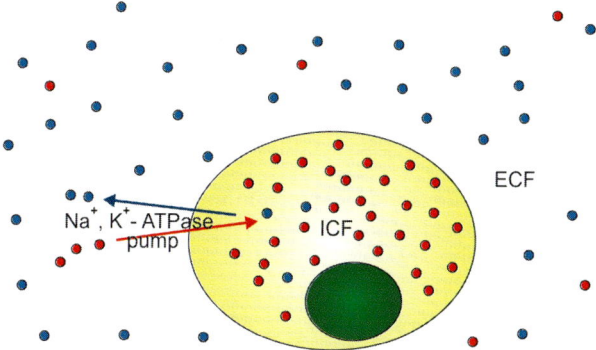

Fig. 29.2: Sodium potassium ATPase pump (blue)—moving potassium (red) into cell and sodium (blue) outside the cell

The fluid intake output chart should be maintained accurately because it helps to decide the correct volume of the replacement fluid. The composition of the infused fluid given depends on what type is lost from the body. For example, if a patient has hemorrhage (bleeding) inside the body or outside, the replacement fluid should be whole blood, blood products or blood substitutes. In a patient with burns, there is loss of plasma and the ideal replacement is plasma. In rare cases, plasma substitutes are used in an emergency if plasma is not available immediately. In patients who have dehydration mainly of ECF compartment, the ideal replacement fluid is normal saline. If the dehydration is severe and is associated with sunken eyeballs, postural hypotension or hypotension and poor skin turgor, there may be intracellular dehydration also. In such cases, normal saline is given first to correct ECF fluid loss followed by 5% dextrose infusions. Dextrose administration is the only means of increasing intracellular water. 5% glucose is isotonic with plasma and can be given safely by IV. The glucose is metabolized by the cell and the intracellular water is replaced successfully. Special precautions are necessary before administering plasma volume expanders (see box).

> **Draw sufficient blood samples for crossmatching before giving plasma volume expanders**
>
> The plasma substitutes may interfere with crossmatching of blood. Therefore, sufficient blood sample for future crossmatching should be drawn before giving plasma substitutes.

MAINTENANCE OF FLUID BALANCE CHART

Fluid balance is the difference between the total 'fluid in' and 'fluid out'. The 'fluid in' consists of oral intake, IV fluid administration and endogenous production of water from metabolism. The oral and IV intake can be measured. The water produced in the body from metabolism of glucose is called endogenous water.

> **Endogenous water from metabolism**
>
> Metabolism of glucose gives rise to carbon dioxide and water. So, the body gains approximately 300–500 ml/day of water from metabolism of glucose. See the equation below:
>
> $$C_6H_{12}O_6 \text{ (Glucose)} + 6O_2 \rightarrow 6CO_2 + 6H_2O \text{ (Water)}$$

The 'fluid out' consists of volume of urine, diarrhea, gastric aspirate and output from drains (if any). These can be accurately measured and charted.

Insensible loss

Insensible fluid loss occurs through skin (sweating) **about 500 ml**, lungs (humidity of expired air) **about 400 ml** and (normal formed) stool **about 100 ml**. The difference between total insensible loss and insensible input is net insensible fluid loss, see the calculation below:

Insensible fluid loss (500 + 400 + 100) – insensible fluid gain (300 to 500)

Net insensible loss 500–700 ml (approximately).

The insensible fluid loss may increase due to physical exercise, sweating, high atmospheric temperature and outdoor activity. In the hospital, fever, extensive wounds, exposure of large raw surfaces (burns) or prolonged exposure to operation light cause increase in insensible fluid loss. Therefore, these factors should be taken into consideration before prescribing the quantity and type of fluids to be administered. A doctor or nurse on duty who is working indoors and having average physical exertion will require about 700 ml of fluid more than the volume of urine. A manual labourer working in the hot climate and undertaking heavy outdoor physical activity may need up to 3 litres or more of fluid intake than the volume of urine. In these examples no disease condition exists. A patient in the ward with fever of 101°F and diarrhea, will need about 1.5 litres of fluid more than the volume of the measured fluid output. Similarly, a patient with nasogastric aspiration will also need the increase in intake to cover the excess volume lost.

In a patient with fluid overload, the volume of fluid must be reduced so that the body will **lose** about 500–800 ml fluid every 24 hours. Patients with oliguria may be prescribed a diuretic to enhance urine output. Combined with restriction of fluid intake, the edema or fluid overload can be effectively controlled.

In the case of very sick patients in ICUs, hourly monitoring of urine output is required. Such patients often have an indwelling catheter draining into a bag. If urine flow meter is not available, the volume of urine in the bag can be measured by **emptying the contents into a measuring cylinder** and **recording the volume every hour**. The markings in the plastic bag may not give accurate values and **all samples must be measured in a graduated container**. The urine flow meter is a transparent graduated container which is incorporated into the regular urine collection bag with a stopcock. By using this, hourly measurement of volume of urine can be made before the urine is drained to the collecting plastic bag (Fig. 29.3).

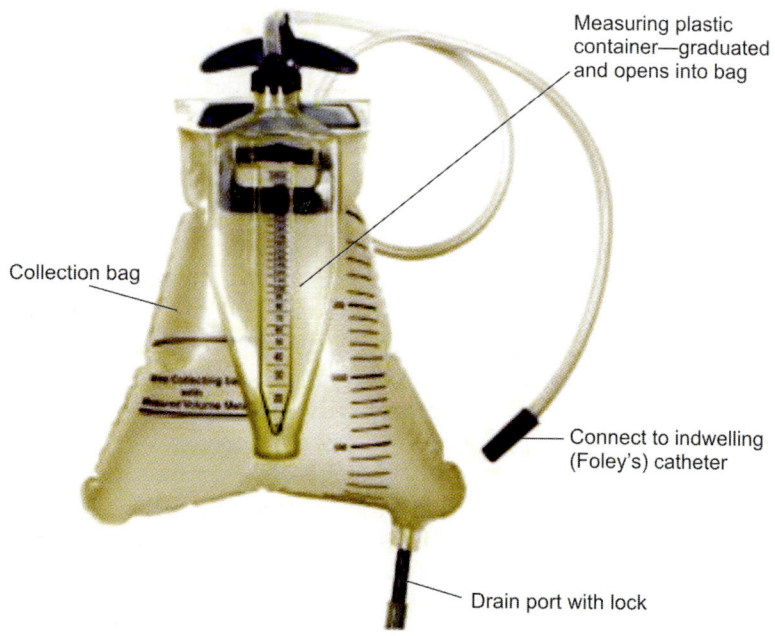

Measuring plastic
container—graduated
and opens into bag

Collection bag

Connect to indwelling
(Foley's) catheter

Drain port with lock

Fig. 29.3: Urine flow meter and urobag

PRECAUTIONS AND CARE OF IV LINES

Earlier, glass bottles were used of intravenous drips. An airway was necessary to permit entry of air into the bottle and smooth flow of the drip. The bubbling of air from the unsterile hospital surroundings may contaminate the 'sterile' IV fluid. So, the bottles are replaced with collapsible pouches. The low density polyethylene (LDPE) and PVC (polyvinyl chloride) pouches are semiopaque and not completely collapsible. In such cases, an airway may have to be used in such a way that the air does not bubble through the fluid. Sometimes, chemicals 'leach' from the poor quality material into the fluid. Good quality pouches are completely collapsible and they do not require any airway. They are crystal clear, completely collapsible and made of polyproplylene. There is no 'leaching' or chemical interaction. Although they may be slightly more expensive, they should be preferred. If the intravenous infusion is maintained as a 'closed system', the chances of contamination are minimised. The infection can occur because of poor technique and during connection and disconnection in a 'closed system'. There-fore, unnecessary connection–disconnection procedures should be avoided. This will help to reduce the rate of infection significantly.

Proper connection of the drip set and further fixing with a "U" bend of the drip set as shown in Fig. 29.4 helps to reduce traction or movement at the connection site between both the canula/vein and canula/drip set junctions. In the event of disconnecting the drip and capping the cannula, only a sterile cap should be used. The cap may be stored in sterilising solution and reused for the same patient only. The cap should never be interchanged between patients. A cap kept on an unsterile surface should not be used. Studies have shown benefit in covering the connection—disconnection sites with antiseptic covers during use or when the cannula is *in situ* and capped (Fig. 29.5).

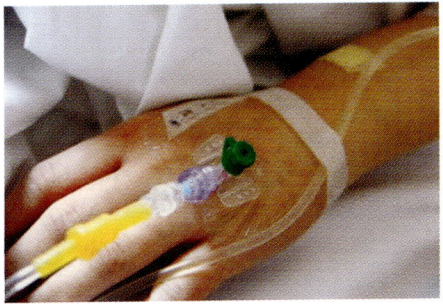

Fig. 29.4: Fixing IV cannula (note the loop in the extension set)

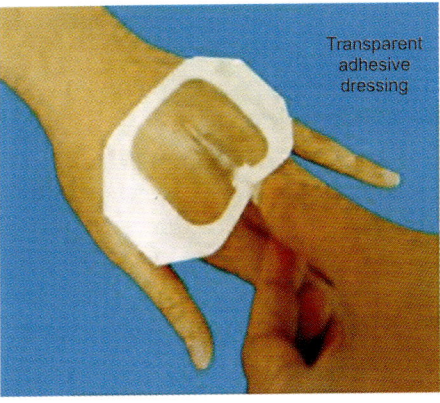

Fig. 29.5: Protection of cannula insertion site (note the connection site is covered well)

Calculating the Rate of Infusion

It is necessary to understand that the fluid administration should be in a timed fashion. If a patient is ordered 3000 ml of fluid per day, it should not be given in 4–6 hours. It should be timed to flow in 24 hours. Too rapid infusion of the whole daily requirement within a few hours will cause fluid overload and cardiovascular strain. If the catheter is well fixed, the patient can have free movement of the hand and do many activities.

Simple calculations are available for finding out the number of drops per minute for giving the fluid in 24 hours. To remember that 1 drop per minute (using regular drip set) gives approximately 100 ml in 24 hours. From this one can easily calculate the number of drops per minute of administering a drip over 24, 12 or 6 hours.

1 drop per minute = 100 ml in 24 hours

Examples:

a. To give 500 ml in 24 hours = 5 drops/min
b. To give 500 ml in 12 hours = 10 drops/min
c. To give 500 ml in 6 hours   = 20 drops/min
d. To give 2500 ml in 24 hours = 25 drops/min
e. To give 3000 ml in 12 hours = 60 drops/min

Now, calculate the number of drops for giving 3500 ml in 12 hours.

(2000 ml in 24 hours is 20 drops per minute. So 2000 ml in 12 hours is 40 drops per minute).

If you are given a challenge as given below, it will be difficult to calculate using the above formula.

Calculate the number of drops for 1000 ml in two and a half hours. For this, a different formula can be used. You can also calculate for different volumes and different time intervals using another simple calculation.

$$\text{Number of drops} = \frac{\text{Volume to be administered (ml)}}{4 \times \text{Time in hours}}$$

So, to give 1000 ml in 2.5 hours, the formula is 1000 divided by 4 = 250 → again divided by 2.5 = 100 drops/min.

More examples:

a. To give 700 ml in 3½ hours—calculate as
$$700/(4 \times 3.5) = 700/14 = 50 \text{ drops/min.}$$

b. To give 1800 ml in 4½ hours—calculate as
$$1800/(4 \times 4.5) = 1800/18 = 100 \text{ drops/min}$$

c. To give 400 ml in 1 hour—calculate as
$$400/(4 \times 1) = 400/4 = 100 \text{ drops/min.}$$

d. To give 640 ml in 4 hours—calculate as
$$640/(4 \times 4) = 640/16 = 40 \text{ drops/min.}$$

The Calculation is Different for Microdrip Set

In the case of microdrops

60 microdrops = 1 ml

30 microdrops/min = 30 ml/hour

or

30 ml/hour = 30 microdrops/min.

Composition of Commonly Used IV Fluids

The intravenous fluids usually used can be divided into 3 main groups:

1. Replacement Fluids (to Replace the Fluid Lost from the Body)

Replacement fluids are used to replace/supplement the fluid that has been lost from the body already. The common fluids used are normal saline (N5), Ringer lactate (RL), dextrose in normal saline (DNS), isolyte G, blood, plasma or colloids.

2. Maintenance Fluids (to Replace the Ongoing Losses)

Maintenance fluids are used to replace the water from the body through lungs, skin, urine and feces which is going on. Since these body fluids are hypotonic and low in sodium, the maintenance fluids are usually 5% dextrose (D5) or half normal saline with dextrose (1/2 NS-D5), isolyte M and isolyte P.

3. Special Fluids

Special fluids are used for special situations. Sodium bicarbonate, potassium chloride, dextrose 25% or 50% are used for special indications. 3% sodium chloride is used in selected cases of acute hyponatremia in ICUs. Colloid solutions are administered with a view to fill up the intravascular space and act as plasma volume expanders. Human albumin, hexa starch or dextran are used as plasma volume expanders.

Replacement Fluids

a. **Normal saline (NS):** It is the most commonly used intravenous fluid in clinical practice. Normal saline is 0.9 % sodium chloride. It contains 0.9 g/100 ml or 9.0 g/L of pure sodium chloride in water. In terms of mmols, the concentration is 154 mmol/L of sodium. Since 0.9% sodium chloride is isotonic with blood, it will not cause hemolysis. Normal saline is distributed mainly ECF compartment. If 1 litre of normal saline is given intravenously, 750 ml will reach the ECF and 250 ml in the intravascular vascular compartment.

It is used when there is loss of water and salt from the body (e.g. diarrhea, vomiting, diabetic ketoacidosis, excessive diuresis, excessive sweating). In hypovolemic shock normal saline is administered to maintain blood pressure until blood transfusion is arranged. (If hypovolemic shock is due to hemorrhage, the ideal replacement is blood.) In hypovolemic shock associated with burns or loss of plasma, the ideal replacement is plasma, albumin or colloids. Normal saline is also used as the main IV fluid in conditions like 'chloride responsive' metabolic alkalosis, acute hypercalcemia or as a diluting agent (vehicle) for administration of other drugs.

It should be avoided or used carefully in patients with fluid overload, cardiac failure, renal failure, hepatic failure, severe hypertension, pre-eclampsia, very young and very old persons and when there is severe hypokalemia (low level of serum potassium).

b. **Ringer lactate (RL): It contains lesser amounts of sodium (120) but contains potassium in approximately the same concentration as normal plasma. It also contains lactate which can be converted in the liver to bicarbonate.** So Ringer lactate is isotonic with blood and is the most physiological fluid. It is distributed in the body similar to normal saline. It is used for correction of diarrhea associated dehydration with hypokalemia and acidosis (small intestinal diarrhea), as fluid replacement in post-operative cases, fractures and burns and cases with severe watery diarrhea. It should be used carefully in liver disease and avoided in acidosis. It cannot be mixed with bank blood or other drugs as vehicle (see the box).

> **Contraindications and cautions while using Ringer lactate**
>
> a. In liver diseases, use of RL may lead to lactic acidosis—accumulation of sodium lactate.
> b. RL is avoided if acidosis is already present (e.g. shock, metformin therapy, severe congestive cardiac failure and severe metabolic acidosis) → worsening of acidosis.
> c. **RL should not be combined with blood through the same IV line or 3-way connector** (calcium in RL will bind to the citrate anticoagulant in the bank blood and cause clotting).
> d. RL cannot be combined with many IV drugs (since calcium may cause reduced efficiency of the drug).

c. **Dextrose normal saline (DNS):** It contains normal saline containing 50 g glucose/litre. DNS is 0.9% sodium chloride (same as normal saline) and 5 g glucose in 100 ml. It is distributed in the body as normal saline. The only advantage is that the glucose in the DNS gives energy (1 g glucose = 3.4 kcal. So 1 litre DNS (50 g glucose) will 170 kcal. So it is used for replacement of extracellular fluid with some energy supply. Correction of dehydration due to vomiting and supply energy. As with NS, it should not be given in fluid overload, severe hypertension and edematous patients. Because of the presence of glucose, it should be given carefully in diabetics and blood sugar monitored. Large volume of DNS may cause hyperglycemia and polyuria even in a non-diabetic person.

d. **Isolyte G:** Otherwise called 'gastric' replacement fluid. Since the gastric juice contains acids combined with approximately 60 mEq/L sodium 100 mEq/L of potassium and 130 mEq/L of chloride. It also contains ammonium which will replace the acid loss. Prolonged vomiting or continuous gastric aspiration may lead to low chloride, high pH and dehydration (hypochloremic metabolic alkalosis). Isolyte G is distributed in the body 50% like NS and 50% like D5. It is used only for replacement of gastric fluid loss and when administration of NH_4Cl is necessary for correction of metabolic alkalosis. It should not be used in hepatic failure since the ammonium is isolyte G which is converted to H^+ ions or unchanged ammonium may worsen hepatic precoma. In renal failure, it may worsen acidosis and increase risk by hyperkalemia.

e. **Isolyte E:** It is an 'Extracellular' replacement solution containing higher concentration of potassium and magnesium. It also contains acetate which is converted to bicarbonate. It provides maximum quantity of bicarbonate as acetate –47 mEq/L in addition to glucose. It is used for correction of dehydration due to diarrhea, correction of associated metabolic acidosis and to maintain ECF volume pre-operatively. It is contraindicated in vomiting, patients with continuous nasogastric aspiration and metabolic alkalosis.

Maintenance Fluids

5% Dextrose, 1/2 NS with dextrose, isolyte M and isolyte P are the commonly used maintenance fluids.

a. **5% Dextrose (D5):** Administration of D5 is equal to administration of water without electrolytes. Since sterile water cannot be given IV because it will cause hemolysis. (Small volumes of sterile distilled water used for diluting certain drugs does not cause hemolysis.) When dextrose 50 g/L is added, we get 5% dextrose and it is nearly istotonic with blood. The glucose is taken up by the tissues and metabolised and water is added to the body's pool. Since D5 contains 50 g anhydrous dextrose/L, 500 ml of 5% dextrose gives 25 g glucose. (Approximate calories intake glucose— 3.4 kcal/g glucose). D5 is distributed uniformly in all body compartments. (60% will be in the intracellular compartment, 30% in interstitial compartment and 10% in intravascular compartments.) D5 is not the appropriate choice of fluid for correcting ECF and intravascular fluid loss. If it is given as the replacement fluid for intravascular volume loss, only 10% of the administered fluid will remain in the intravascular compartment. It is used to prevent and treat dehydration (due to poor intake or excessive water loss), pre/postoperative fluid replacement, as vehicle for administering drugs, to prevent starvation ketosis and correct high serum sodium (hypernatremia) due to excessive sweating/diabetes insipidus. It is contraindicated in cerebral edema, following neurosurgical procedures, ischemic stroke, hypovolemic shock and hyponatremia. During administration, blood sugar, K^+, Mg^{++} and phosphates are monitored. If higher concentration of glucose like 25% or 50% are given through peripheral vein, it may cause thrombophlebitis. Blood transfusion and D5 should not be given through the same IV line because hemolysis may occur.

b. **Half normal saline with 5% dextrose (1/2 NS-D5):** In contrast with DNS, 1/2 NS-5D contains only 50% of the sodium chloride compared to NS and 50 g/L of dextrose. It is useful to supply calories and water with less salt. It is preferred in pediatric patients who need more water than salt. The distribution within body fluid compartments is 75% as 5D and 25% as NS. This is the ideal maintenance fluid for children and postoperative patients. It is also used as maintenance fluid in adults. It should not be given if the patient has hyponatremia or dehydration which will cause loss of salt since the salt content is only 50% of NS.

c. **Isolyte M:** It is a type of maintenance fluid with dextrose and is hypotonic, low in Na and rich in potassium. It is used in patients with hypokalemia. **It should be used only in patients who have normal renal function and good urine output.** It also supplies energy and corrects acidosis. It is distributed within the body mostly in intracellular compartment. It does not significantly improve the intravascular volume. It can be used in patients with dehydration and hypokalemia. It should not be used for renal failure and low serum sodium (hyponatremia).

d. **Isolyte P:** This is the maintenance fluid used in children. Children need more water and regular supply of electrolytes, calories with bicarbonate. 1 Litre of isolyte P contains 50 g glucose, sodium lactate, potassium chloride, magnesium chloride and dibasic potassium phosphate. It is distributed similar to D5 and is used in children and those with diabetes insipidus. (The distribution is similar to D5. Hence it does not increase intravascular volume significantly.) Hyponatremia, renal failure, hypovolemic shock and oliguric patients should not be given this type of fluid. Rapid administration is avoided.

Special Fluids

The special fluids are usually available as ampoules or in small volume sterile pouches. These special fluids are usually added to respective IV fluids as decided by the clinician and administered in a dilute form. Care is taken to avoid a mixture of non-compatible fluids/solution (see the box).

Examples of incompatible combinations

a. If sodium bicarbonate and any calcium containing fluid are mixed or given through the same infusion set, needle or vein, precipitation of insoluble calcium carbonate (white precipitate) will occur **immediately**.

b. If calcium is added to the bank blood, it will neutralize the anti-coagulant effect of citrate in the blood and **cause clotting of blood in the blood bag or drip set**.

c. Some drugs are incompatible when mixed with some of the commonly used IV fluids. Therefore, great care is taken to avoid such incidents.

d. Many drugs should not be mixed with calcium containing fluids.

e. For most drugs, the ideal vehicle for dilution will be specified in the pamphlet supplied with the packing.

a. **Sterile sodium bicarbonate:** It is usually available as 25 ml ampoules containing 7.5 % solution. 25 ml contains 22.5 mEq each of sodium and bicarbonate. It is a very useful drug in emergencies like cardiac arrest, hyperkalemia and shock. In cardiac arrest, sodium bicarbonate, 100 ml, is given intravenously as a bolus as a part of resuscitation (see the box).

How is sodium bicarbonate beneficial in cardiac arrest?

When cardiac arrest occurs, lactic acidosis develops and the acidosis is neutralised immediately by administration of the alkali-sodium bicarbonate.

It is also used sometimes in treatment of shock, for the emergency management of hyperkalemia with acidosis in a patient with renal failure, metabolic acidosis and in forced alkaline diuresis.

What is forced alkaline diuresis?

Forced alkaline diuresis is administration of IV fluid with a slightly alkaline pH. The volume administered depends on the output. A diuretic is often given to increase the output. Some drugs are excreted in the urine better if the urine is alkaline. Thus, forced alkaline diuresis helps to increase the excretion of some drugs/toxins from the body through the kidney.

It should be diluted and given in 1/2 NS-D5 as infusion. If it is added to NS, it may cause sodium overload and pulmonary edema. It may precipitate hypocalcemic tetany, and worsen hypokalemia. It should not be mixed with calcium containing fluids or ionotopic drugs like non-adrenalin, dopamine or dobutamine. The infusion should be given only through a large vein if given in undiluted form. It should be used carefully in fluid overloaded states and hypertension because of the sodium content.

b. **Potassium chloride (KCl):** Sterile potassium chloride is usually available in 10 ml ampoules containing 1.5 g KCl (20 mEq potassium). So 1 ml of KCl = 150 mg KCl = 2 mmol. Important caution for using IV potassium chloride (see the box).

Precaution while using intravenous potassium

Potassium chloride should **NEVER** be given as a bolus injection.
It will cause **Cardiac Arrest.**
It must be diluted and given **as a Drip** in a controlled fashion only.

Potassium is an intracellular cation. The blood level is maintained in the range of 3.5 to 5.0 mg and this is essential for normal neuromuscular function. High serum potassium may lead to a series of ECG changes leading to cardiac arrest if not diagnosed and treated early. KCl may be added to potassium poor IV fluids as part of maintenance fluid therapy. In cases with hypokalemia, KCl may be added to the appropriate fluid and administered as a controlled infusion monitoring ECG and blood level of potassium.

c. **Hypertonic sodium chloride (3% NaCl):** Hypertonic sodium chloride is available as 3% and 5%. However, 3% NaCl, containing 30 g sodium in 1 liter water is used clinically. It contains 513 mmol sodium/L and has a high osmolality –1030 mOsm/kg. (5% sodium chloride is not commonly available). Hypertonic sodium chloride is used in severe symptomatic hyponatremia with serum sodium <115 mmol/L. Only if the patient has severe acute onset of hyponatremia with early neurologic symptoms or impending convulsions, hypertonic sodium chloride is used. It is useful in patients who have very low sodium and chloride, or those who have low serum sodium due to excess water retention by the body. Rapid infusions to correct sodium >10 mmol/day are harmful. It should not be used in mild asymptomatic hyponatremia, or administered rapidly. It should be used only in ICU set up.

Remember

1000 ml of 3% NaCl gives approximately 500 mmol Na (actual 513).

or

2 ml of 3% NaCl gives approximately 1 mmol sodium.

or

1 ml of 3% NaCl gives approximately 0.5 mmol sodium.

d. Colloids: Fluids which contain larger molecules (colloids) remain within the vascular system if given through intravenous route. So, they help to increase the volume in the intravascular compartment. If blood or plasma are not available and the patient is progressing to shock, it may be necessary to use plasma volume expanders to maintain circulatory fluid volume. The effect of plasma volume expanders is usually temporary and lasting for less than 24 hours. The appropriate replacement fluid must be administered in the meantime.

1. Human albumin is obtained by separation from pooled screened plasma of blood donors. Intravenous human albumin is available as 5% in 500 or 1000 ml containers containing 50 g albumin/L. 20% is available in 100 ml bottles containing 20 g albumin. It can be used not only for replacing albumin, but also in a patient with hypoproteinemia with edema which is resistant to diuretics. By giving albumin intravascular oncotic pressure increases and the fluid from the ECF is drawn into intravascular space. This helps to increase intravascular volume by an additional 300–400 ml and the fluid can be eliminated by the kidneys. The effect of IV albumin is temporary and may last for 48–72 hours only. Albumin is also used as replacement of protein in patients, undergoing plasmaphresis. Rapid infusion of albumin may lead to circulatory overload or pulmonary edema.

2. Dextrans are used for expanding plasma volume in emergencies. They are useful in battle fields or ambulances during transport of the patient to a hospital. Both low molecular weight –40 (MW 40,000) and high molecular weight dextrans 70 (MW 70,000) are available. Dextran 40 is 10% solution. The maximum first dose is 1000 ml during the first 24 hours. It may be repeated at a dose of maximum of 500 ml on the second day. It produces rapid volume expansion of intravascular compartment and helps to prevent thromboembolism, improves microcirculation and minimises sludging in blood vessels. It is useful in impending shock or early shock. Dextron 70 has slower onset of action but prolonged duration. The important side effects are acute kidney injury (AKI) and hypersensitivity. Use of dextrans may interfere with blood grouping and

crossmatching. Therefore, adequate blood samples may be drawn for grouping and future crossmatching for blood transfusions. It should not be used if the patient is oliguric, has AKI, cardiac disease/failure, dehydration, active bleeding or chronic liver disease.

3. *Gelatin polymer (haemaccel):* Gelatin polymers are obtained from degraded gelatin. It contains NaCl –145 mmol, $CaCl_2$ –6.25 mmol (12.5 g), KCl –5.1 mmol with degraded gelatin polypeptides (polygelin) –35 g in 1 litre water. Infusions are available in 500 ml sterile pouches. It is contraindicated in patients who exhibit a generalized allergic tendency. It should be used very cautiously in patients with cardiac and renal failure. The actions are similar to dextran. However, it does not interfere with blood coagulation, grouping or crossmatching.

4. *Hydroxyethyl starch:* It is a colloidal suspension of starch derivative (nonionic) in saline. It is used as a volume expander. However, since the complications like acute kidney injury (which may occur even in a delayed fashion, higher chances of hypersensitivity, cardiac arrhythmias, bronchospasm and pulmonary edema, it is not commonly used in most ICUs. It may also cause disturbances in blood coagulation. Patients with intracranial bleeding should not be given this. Because of the chances of accumulation in the body, it should not be given for more than 24 hours. Many countries are considering a ban on the use of this.

30

Normal and Abnormal and Electrolyte Homeostasis

R Kasi Visweswaran

The body is able to control the composition of body fluids by adjusting the intake and excretion of water and electrolytes under normal conditions. The thirst mechanism controls the intake of water. If someone does not take enough water, the antidiuretic hormone (ADH or vasopressin) is secreted from the posterior pituitary gland. This acts on the kidneys and make the kidneys reabsorb more water and produce less urine. On the other hand, if a person takes excessive quantities of liquids, this hormone is suppressed and the kidney forms more urine and the excess fluid is excreted as urine. We can experience this in everyday life. On a hot day, we feel more thirsty and drink more water, whereas on a cold day, the water we drink is automatically less because we do not feel thirsty. The kidneys are able to excrete or retain salt as required by the body. Similarly, the kidneys and other hormone systems in the body are able to regulate the excretion of electrolytes like potassium, calcium, magnesium, and phosphates to maintain the blood level in the normal range. This is called homeostasis. The homeostasis can be disturbed when abnormal intake or excretion of these substances occurs or in diseases.

The homeostasis of water and sodium is closely linked. In order to maintain the water and sodium homeostasis, the fluid intake and output must be approximately equal. The intake includes the food or intravenous fluids and the output represents the volume of urine. In disease conditions, vomitus and diarrheal fluid should also be calculated as output. The 'insensible' (endogenous) water production from the metabolism and the 'insensible' water loss cannot be measured. However, approximate insensible loss can be assessed depending on presence of fever, temperature of the surroundings (ambient), physical activity or other factors. The water balance is also maintained by regulating the urine output.

SODIUM AND WATER HOMEOSTASIS

Sodium concentration in the ECF is much higher than ICF. The average normal salt intake is approximately 6 gm. Depending on the need of the body, the excretion of salt is regulated by the kidney. When a person is dehydrated, more salt is reabsorbed and urine will contain very low quantity of sodium. Otherwise, urinary sodium will be higher. Usually, only 0 to 2% of the filtered sodium is excreted in the urine. Hormones like aldosterone, atrial natriuretic peptide and hydrocortisone regulate sodium reabsorption by the kidney.

Abnormal conditions causing loss of water from the body are through external or internal hemorrhage, GI losses (vomiting/diarrhea/fistulas), sweating, or loss into 'third space'. The third space is neither in the ICF compartment nor in the ECF compartment. The fluid is drawn to the 'third space' firstly from the ECF compartment. The event which causes shifting of the fluid into the 'third' space are mentioned below (see the box).

Event	Sequestration of fluid
Examples:	
1. Obstruction to gastrointestinal tract	Bowel lumen
2. Severe burns	Subcutaneous tissue
3. Acute pancreatitis	Retroperitoneal space
4. Peritonitis	Peritoneal cavity
5. Cirrhosis of liver	Peritoneal cavity
6. Nephrotic syndrome	Pleura/peritoneum

As the abnormalities of water and sodium are closely interlinked, they are discussed together under the following headings.

Hypovolemia: A condition where there is combined salt and water loss (loss of water more than the intake).

Hypervolemia: This condition occurs when there is water intake more than total output in those with cardiac, renal or hepatic disease.

Hyponatremia: A condition where the serum sodium is <135 mmol/L (common problem in hospitalized patients).

Hypernatremia: Hypernatremia is defined as plasma sodium >145 mmol/L (occurs commonly in ICUs).

Hypovolemia: Occurs when there is excessive water loss from the body causing reduction of ECF volume. Common causes are given in the box.

Source of water loss Examples:	Disease or condition
Kidneys	Diabetes insipidus, uncontrolled diabetes mellitus Diuretics, salt losing kidney diseases.
Skin	Heat exhaustion/heat stroke
GI system	Diarrhea/biliary, pancreatic or intestinal fistula
Resp. system	Prolonged artificial ventilation
Blood/plasma	Hemorrhage, burns, severe infections (necrotizing fasciitis)

Dehydration and hypovolemia are common problems. Prompt identification and correct treatment can successfully correct the dehydration. When ECF volume reduces, the patient may develop postural hypotension and tachycardia followed by persistant hypotension. The kidneys try to reabsorb sodium and water to the maximum possible. So, the patient may develop oliguria with low urinary sodium (< 20 mmol/L). When dehydration is more severe, the skin **turgor** is lost, the mucous membranes become dry, the eyeballs appear sunken and the **jugular venous pressure** is low and the pulsations may not be seen even in lying position. Later, patient may faint when he tries to stand up due to fall in blood pressure in erect position (postural hypotension). Later on the patient may go to shock. When we touch the patient, he may feel 'cold and clammy' (see the box).

'Turgor'

Turgor means elasticity—'skin turgor' means ability of the skin to resume th original position when it is pinched and released. For example, when the skin over forehead is pinched and released, it retains the original shape without any delay. In a patient with severe dehydration, it takes more time pinched skin to resume original shape. Skin turgor is seen best in skin directly over a bone. (Examples: Forehead, back of forearm or sternum.)

'Clammy'

'Clammy' means moist, sticky, cold and gives an unpleasant sensation for the examiner when he touches.

Jugular venous pulsations

The pulsations in the jugular vein can be seen as wavy pulsation in the root of the neck when a normal person is lying down.

In a patient with severe dehydration, the pulsation may not be visible even in the lying position.

If the patient has gross fluid overload or cardiac failure, the jugular pulsations will be visible in the neck even in sitting position.

A proper history and physical examination often help to identify the cause and severity of ECF volume contraction. The treatment is to restore ECF volume deficit. The basic fluid required is **normal saline**. Later, appropriate changes may be necessary depending on the type of fluid lost. Monitoring can be done by improvement in blood pressure, skin turgor, jugular venous pressure, normalization of pulse rate and overall clinical status. CVP or pulmonary capillary wedge pressure monitoring can be undertaken in ICUs in serious conditions.

HYPERVOLEMIA

Hypervolemia does not occur in a normal person because the kidneys are capable of excreting nearly 10 liters of extra fluid in a day. Hypervolemia may occur if there is cardiac, liver or renal disease associated with high fluid intake. The patient may have pedal edema or ascites or elevated jugular venous pressure.

In cardiac disease, the patient will have elevated JVP with pedal edema and pulmonary congestion. If there is left heart (ventricular) failure, there may be pulmonary edema and orthopnea (inability to lie flat in bed). If there is right ventricular failure, there will be combination of increased JVP, liver enlargement and pedal edema. In renal disease, facial puffiness in the morning and dependant pedal edema by evening occur in early stages. In later stages, these patients may have persistent pedal edema, generalized edema or associated with effusion in pleural, pericardial and abdominal cavities. This is called the stage of 'anasarca'. If hypervolemia is due to liver disease, ascites is the most important manifestation. Children or adults who have severe hypoalbuminemia due to nutritional causes may also develop dependant edema. Children with kwashiorkor (a condition of severe malnutrition with deficiency of proteins and calories), the lower half of the body may be grossly edematous but the upper half of the body may not show edema.

Hypervolemia is treated by regulating fluid intake, correction of causative illness and use of diuretics. In cases with hypo-albuminemia (chronic liver disease, nutritional deficiency or nephrotic syndrome), albumin infusions may bring about tempo-rary relief. In chronic renal disease, regulation of fluid intake is the most useful method.

HYPONATREMIA

There are 2 conditions where the serum sodium may be **falsely low**. In patients with hyperlipidemia or hyperproteinemia, the serum sodium may appear to be low even though the actual sodium concentration plasma is normal. This is called **pseudohyponatremia.** If plasma sodium is assessed by special tests (using ion specific electrodes), it will be normal. When substances like glucose, mannitol or glycine are administered, there is movement of water from ICF to ECF. More water in ECF dilutes the ECF compartment and reduces Na^+ concentration. This is called **translocational hyponatremia**. It may be present when hypertonic glucose (parental hyperalimentation), mannitol (for reducing brain edema) or glycine (for bladder irrigation in transurethral reaction of prostate gland) are used.

Classification of True Hyponatremia

True hyponatremia is classified into:

a. *Hyponatremia with ECF* volume depletion: hypovolemic hyponatremia.

b. *Hyponatremia with ECF* volume expansion: hypervolemic hyponatremia

c. *Hyponatremia with* normal *ECF* volume: euvolemic hyponatremia

In **hypovolemic hyponatremia**, there is a loss of sodium and water but sodium loss is greater than water loss. The loss can be through kidneys, extrarenal causes like vomiting, diarrhea, burns, muscle injury, pancreatitis or loss into body compartments. It is possible to differentiate between renal and extrarenal losses by checking the urinary sodium. In renal loss, the urinary sodium will be high (see the box).

Urine sample for sodium estimation

Urine sample for sodium estimation should be taken before administering a diuretic. Otherwise, the results may give a false high value.

In **hypervolemic hyponatremia** there is increase in total body sodium and water but the serum level is 'low' because of relatively more water retention. This is also called 'dilutional hyponatremia'. The common conditions associated with this are nephrotic syndrome, cirrhosis of liver and cardiac failure. Since the kidneys retain salt instead of excreting it, the urinary sodium may be low (<20 mmol/L).

In **euvolemic hyponatremia**, the ECF volume is normal but the sodium is low. The commonest condition causing this is the **S**yndrome of **I**nappropriate **ADH** (**SIADH**) secretion. Other conditions like deficiency of thyroid hormone (hypothyroidism), adrenocortical hormone deficiency (Addison's disease), head injury, physical or emotional stress and drugs can cause similar condition. When there is excessive ADH, the kidney to reabsorb more water (antidiuresis) which results in water retention. There is dilutional hyponatremia and increased water in ICF and ECF. These patients are usually not edematous but there is sodium loss (natriuresis) and water retention. The treatment of SIADH, is by restriction of water and promoting water loss. SIADH may be associated with some carcinomas (lung, duodenum, pancreas), CNS diseases (encephalitis, meningitis, psychosis, stroke, tumor, abscess, trauma, hemorrhage), lung diseases, AIDS and use of some drugs (nicotine, chlorpropamide, clofibrate, cyclophosphamide, NSAIDs, antipsychotics, antidepressants).

SYMPTOMS AND SIGNS OF HYPONATREMIA

Symptoms and signs of hyponatremia depend on whether it occurs suddenly or gradually. If it develops within 48 hrs, it is called 'acute'. Acute hyponatremia is associated with cerebral edema and neurologic symptoms occur (Table 30.1).

If hyponatremia develops gradually (>48 hrs), the body adapts to the low sodium and there is no cerebral edema and the patient

Table 30.1: Symptoms and signs of acute hyponatremia

Symptoms	Signs
Lethargy	Abnormal sensorium
Disorientation	Depressed tendon reflex
Muscle cramps	Hyperthermia
Anorexia/nausea	Coma
Agitation	Seizures

is asymptomatic. Rapid correction of asymptomatic chronic hyponatremia may lead to even permanent brain damage called 'osmotic demyelination syndrome' or 'Central pontine myelinolysis'. In this condition, there is cell shrinkage and damage to regions of the brainstem called pons.

Mild asymptomatic hyponatremia may need no specific treatment. If there is ECF volume contraction, sodium containing fluids—oral rehydration solution, drinks with salt can be given by mouth. In selected cases intravenous infusion of normal saline may be necessary to correct the ECF volume deficit. Infusion may be continued when ECF volume deficiency is corrected. Patients with hyponatremia with volume expansion (nephritic/hepatic/cardiac edema) are treated with restricting sodium and water combined with potassium supplementation if hypokalemia is present. By using loop diuretics water and sodium are lost, only the sodium that is lost is replaced and water intake is restricted. Potassium level should be maintained. In euvolemic hyponatremia due to condition like SIDH, water restriction is the main focus of treatment.

HYPERNATREMIA

Hypernatremia may occur due to sodium gain or water loss. Increased sodium stimulates the thirst center. The thirst will make the patient drink water. Hypernatremia does not occur if the thirst mechanism is alright and the person is able to drink water when he wants. If the patient is in the ICU and intake of water is regulated by the staff under the direction of the doctor, the patient may not get water when he is thirsty. Usually, there is dehydration in ICF compartment. Hypernatremia is classified as:

- Hypovolemic hypernatremia
- Hypervolemic hypernatremia and
- Euvolemic hypernatremia

Hypovolemic hypernatremia (high serum sodium with decreased body water): It occurs when there is water loss but no sodium loss. It can occur due to problems in the kidney [renal causes such as use of diuretics and conditions of polyuria (output >3000 ml in 24 hours]. It can be due to problems not related to kidney (extra-renal causes such as diarrhea, heat exposure, sun stroke, severe exercise, burns, or hyperglycemia). Confused patients who refuse food or fluids and those in coma may develop hypernatremia. Most cases of hypernatremia are due to water deficit.

Hypervolemic hyponatremia (high serum sodium with increased body water): Hypervolemic hypernatremia occurs due to incorrect use of hypertonic saline or sodium bicarbonate infusions. Patients have ECF volume expansion, edema, pulmonary congestion or raised jugular venous pressure.

Euvolemic hypernatremia (high serum sodium with normal body water): Diabetes insipidus (DI) is an important illness which may be associated with euvolemic hypernatremia. It may also occur due to excess water loss from the body through sweating, fever or other hypercatabolic states. In diabetes insipidus (DI), there is profound polyuria. It may be either due to central DI (deficiency of antidiuretic hormone production) or due to the kidneys not responding to the normal production of ADH.

Hypernatremia is treated by preventing water loss and correcting water deficit. If the hypernatremia is acute (<48 hours), it has to be corrected promptly. Treatment of hypernatremia is by water administration. The safest route of water administration is oral or tube feeding. In rare situations, it may be necessary to supplement water by IV route. Intravenous 5% glucose drip is isotonic with blood and does not cause hemolysis of RBCs. After IV administration, the glucose is metabolized, the body gets pure water (without sodium).

POTASSIUM HOMEOSTASIS

Potassium (K^+) is a cation. It is present mainly in the intracellular compartment (150 mmol/L). The whole body contains about 3500 mmol K^+. The serum K^+ concentration is maintained in a narrow range of 3.5 to 5.0 mmol/L and is important for normal neuromuscular function. The diet provides between 40 and 120 mmols which is almost completely absorbed from the GIT to reach the plasma. Under the influence of insulin and by the action of Na^+, K^+-ATPase pump, it moves into the intracellular compartment. Most of the K^+ is excreted through the urine. The K^+ excretion in the kidney is regulated by the hormone aldosterone which is secreted from the adrenal cortex. When serum K^+ level is high, more K^+ will be excreted and when it is low, more will be retained. Aldosterone causes increased K^+ excretion in the urine. Therefore, conditions associated with aldosterone excess (hyperaldosteronism) cause hypokalemia. The urinary loss of K^+ is about 20–25 mmol. The decrease in serum K^+ is not proportional to total body's potassium loss. The patient may have lost $\approx$ 250–300 mmol/K before serum level decreases by 1 mmol/L. The loss of K^+ from various body fluid loss is shown below:

Sweat	$\rightarrow$	10 mmol/L (volume of sweat may be variable)
Stool	$\rightarrow$	100 mmol/day
Diarrhea	$\rightarrow$	**40–50 mmol/L**
Renal	$\rightarrow$	10 mmol/day

The two important abnormalities relating to K^+ homeostasis are hypokalemia and hyperkalemia. Both conditions are common and can cause life-threatening complications.

Hypokalemia is defined as serum K^+ below 3.5 mmol/L. Spurious hypokalemia may occur if there is extreme leucocytosis. True hypokalemia occurs due to loss of K^+ from the body. The loss can be due to renal or extra-renal losses (see the box).

Urinary loss of K^+	Nonrenal loss of K^+
a. Diuretic therapy	a. Vomiting/continuous NG suction
b. Cushing's syndrome (glucocorticoid excess)	b. Ureterosigmoidostomy—artificial opening of ureter to intestine or artificial bladder using intestine
c. Chronic interstitial nephritis	c. Alcoholism
	d. Hypokalemia periodic paralysis
	e. Diarrhea/laxative abuse
	f. Metabolic alkalosis and

K^+ is important for proper functioning of nerves and muscle (neuromuscular function). Patients with hypokalemia may have extreme weakness, paralysis, respiratory failure, paralytic ileus, tetany or hepatic coma. The ECG may show the changes in severe hypokalemia—the T wave becomes smaller and disappears, U wave appears and ST segment sags down as shown in Fig. 30.1.

Mild to moderate asymptomatic hypokalemia is managed with avoidance of precipitating factors and increasing dietary K^+ intake. If necessary, potassium chloride solution (which contains 15 mmol K^+ per 10 ml) may be given orally in diluted form every 4–6 hours. Potassium is also available as slow release capsule contains 8 mmol of K^+/capsule. Potassium therapy should be monitored by blood tests and ECG. In severe hypokalemia with muscle paralysis, myopathy respiratory failure, infusion of potassium chloride are

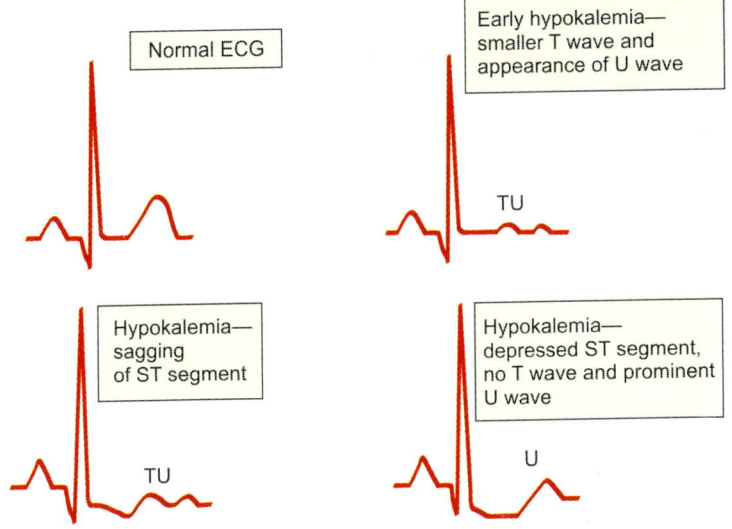

Fig. 30.1: ECG changes in hypokalemia

used to tide over the crisis. When K⁺ falls from 3.5 to 3 mmol/L, the body may have lost 150–200 mmol and if it has fallen from 3 to 2 mmol, the deficit may be 200–400 mmol or even more. Potassium chloride must **never be given as bolus injection**. It should be diluted in dextrose or NS and given as a **slow intravenous drip** only.

Hyperkalemia is diagnosed when serum potassium exceeds 5.5 mmol/L. If there is moisture in the collecting syringe or sample bottle, destruction (lysis) of RBCs may occur in the sample and the lab may give high K⁺ report. Other conditions causing false high values are extreme thrombocyosis, leucoytosis or prolonged tourniquet application before drawing the blood sample. This is called **pseudohyperkalemia** and is never accompanied by ECG changes. The causes of acute hyperkalemia are enumerated in Table 30.2.

When many factors are present in the same patient, the severity of hyperkalemia will be more, e.g. diabetic with renal failure and aldosterone deficiency taking pain killers is predisposed to severe hyperkalemia.

Usually there is no specific symptoms for hyperkalemia. Vague GI symptoms, weakness, constipation may occur. Often the diagnosis is made from the blood test or ECG. Serial changes in ECG in hyperkalemia are shown in Fig. 30.2.

Table 30.2: Acute hyperkalemia	
A. *Shifting of intracellular K⁺ to ECF*	B. *Defects in excretion of K⁺ by the kidney*
i. Insulin deficiency	i. Renal failure
ii. Beta blocker therapy	ii. K⁺ sparing diuretics
iii. Metabolic acidosis	iii. Drugs acting over renin angiotensin system
iv. Rhabdo myolosis (severe muscle injury)	iv. NSAID use
v. Drug actions	v. Addison's diseases (adrenocortical deficiency)
	vi. Type 4 renal tubular acidosis

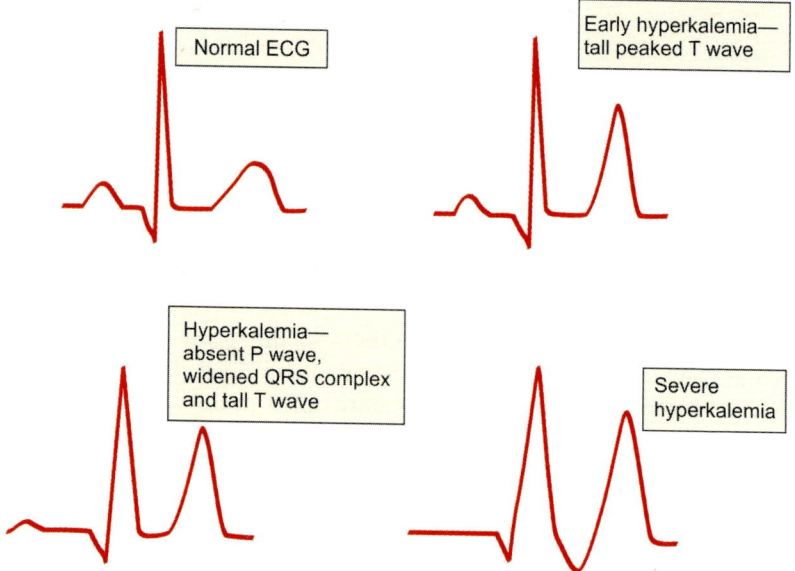

Fig. 30.2: ECG changes in hyperkalemia

If serum K⁺ is <6, ECG changes and neuromuscular abnormalities are not present, hyperkalemia can be managed by reducing dietary K⁺ intake or withholding the offending drug (often ACE inhibitors, beta blockers, potassium sparing diuretics, NSAIDs or potassium supplements). If serum K⁺ is >6, ECG changes and neuromuscular abnormalities are present, hyperkalemia should be treated as a medical emergency. The steps in the emergency management are:

   i. Calcium gluconate— 10–30 ml of 10% solution (available as ampoules) is given as a very **slow intravenous infusion (under cardiac monitoring,** if available). Calcium administration helps to prevent ventricular fibrillation and cardiac arrest by stabilizing the myocardium. The protective action will stop as soon as the IV infusion is over.

  ii. As the calcium administration is going on slowly, another team organizes IV infusion of 10%. Glucose with 10 units crystalline (plain/actrapid) insulin added and the infusion is given at 100 ml/hr for 2 hours (about 24 drops per minute will give 100 ml/hr). Administration of glucose with insulin helps to move (shift) the potassium from ECF to ICF compartment.

 iii. Use of terbutaline or salbutamol 10 mg in 4 ml normal saline can be given by nebulisation. This also helps to shift the K^+ into the cell (ICF).

 iv. If the patient has acidosis, use of sodium bicarbonate IV will also help to shift the K^+ into the cell.

Excretion of K^+ from the body occurs only through urine or feces. In hyperkalemia due to kidney disease, only potassium exchange resins and dialysis can remove K^+ from the body. 15 gm of potassium exchange resin (kayexelate) is given orally (with 30 ml sorbitol or mixed with food) every 4–6 hours. It can also be given as retention enema of 45 gm with 70% sorbitol and 100 ml water. In the intestine, the resin will exchange K^+ for sodium. Later, the resin containing the K^+ is excreted. Both hemodialysis and peritoneal dialysis can remove K^+ effectively from the blood.

CALCIUM HOMEOSTASIS

Calcium has a very important role to play in cardiac contraction, hormone secretion, blood coagulation and neuromuscular actions. The body contains nearly 1.4 kg calcium out of which 99% in the bones. In the blood and tissues, calcium is either bound to albumin ($\simeq$ 40%), free (ionized form about 50–55%) or complexed with phosphate, bicarbonate, citrate, lactate, etc (< 5%). The ionised form of calcium is the active form and is more important than total serum calcium. Since 40% calcium is bound to albumin, in patients with hypoalbuminemia, the total serum calcium may be low although the ionic calcium is normal. Serum calcium level is maintained in the narrow range of 9 to 11 mg/dL (ionic calcium 4.5 to 5.5 mg/dl) and is controlled by parathyroid hormone, active vitamin D, intestines, bones and kidney. Hypocalcemia stimulates PTH and it acts on the bones to reabsorb calcium and correct the blood level. In hypercalcemia, the body tries to excrete more calcium in urine.

Calculating corrected calcium

In patients with hypoalbuminemia, the blood level obtained from the laboratory may be falsely low. Therefore, it is necessary to correct the serum calcium values depending on the degree of hypoalbuminemia.

When serum albumin is <4 gm/dl, for every 1 gm/dl reduction in serum albumin, add 0.8 mg/dl calcium to the laboratory value to get the corrected calcium level.

Example: If the patient has serum calcium level of 7.5 and serum albumin of 2.0 gm/dl, (reduction of albumin 2 gm/dl below 4.0 gm/dl). Therefore, add 1.6 mg/dl to the available laboratory value.

So, the **corrected serum calcium** will be **7.5 + 1.6 = 9.1 mg/dl.**

Hypercalcemia is a condition where the serum calcium is **>11.5 mg/dl.** The serum calcium increases in conditions associated with increased secretion of parathyroid hormone (hyperparathyroidism), excessive use of vitamin A or vitamin D, prolonged immobilization or use of drugs (thiazide diuretics, theophylline, lithium and calcium).

Signs and symptoms of hypercalcemia depend on the severity and rate of onset. Symptoms due to the primary disease will be present in early stages, there may be nausea, loss of apetite, constipation or sluggishness of central nervous system activity and reflexes. Later, alteration in mental state, seizures and coma may develop. Severe symptoms occur only when the serum calcium level is over 17 mg/dl. The ECG may show prolongation of QT interval.

Treatment includes hydration to correct the associated extracellular fluid volume deficit, avoidance of calcium, vitamin A, vitamin D and other causative drugs and treatment of the primary condition.

Hypocalcemia

In hypocalcemia, the corrected serum calcium is **less than 8.5 mg/dl.** The result of serum calcium should be interpreted only with the corresponding blood report of serum albumin. In conditions associated with hypoalbuminemia like nephrotic syndrome, liver disease, and malnutrition, the measured serum calcium may be lower.

Hypocalcemia occurs in acute or chronic renal failure, vitamin D or Mg deficiency, acute pancreatitis, hypoparathyroidism, pseudohypoparathyroidism, malnutrition and respiratory alkalosis. Administration of calcium free albumin or repeated blood transfusions (citrate infusion) can lead to hypocalcemia in hospitalized patients.

Repeated blood transfusions and hypocalcemia

When a patient receives multiple blood transfusions, large dose of citrate (anticoagulant) enters the body.

Excessive citrate not only causes hypocalcemia but also bleeding tendency. Therefore, calcium infusions should be given to the patient receiving multiple transfusions.

Calcium through a separate intravenous line.

(*Note:* If calcium is added to the blood bag, the blood will clot in the bag)

Early symptoms of hypocalcemia are muscle cramps, tetany, impaired mental capacity, personality changes and depression. Dementia or seizures may occur in severe hypocalcemia. The ECG may show prolongation of QT segment or arrhythmia.

Treatment depends on the cause. For less severe cases, oral calcium supplements—calcium carbonate 1gm thrice daily is given combined with active vitamin D (1,25-dihydroxycholecalciferol) 0.25 to 0.5 microgram daily. 10% calcium gluconate 10 ml is given slowly at 0.5 ml/minute for tetany or cardiac arrhythmia. Calcium should not be given rapidly IV since it can cause cardiac arrest. If the symptoms do not subside, 8 ampoules of calcium gluconate (80 ml) is diluted in 500 ml of 5% glucose and given at approximately 25 drops per minute (about 6–8 hours).

DISORDERS OF PHOSPHATE METABOLISM

Phosphorus and calcium are the main ingredients of the bone. About 85% of the phosphorus in the body forms the part of the bone. The phosphorus in the blood and tissues is very important for cellular metabolism and functions. Phosphate is present in the DNA, RNA and adenosine tri-phosphate (ATP). The cells get the energy from the conversion of ATP to adenosine di-phosphate (ADP). In the blood, phosphorus is present as inorganic phosphate **(3–4.5 mg/dl in adults and 4–7 mg/dl in children).**

Hyperphosphatemia

Defined as serum phosphate level of >5 mg/dl in adults and >7 mg/dl in children. It occurs due to excessive intake, defective excretion or other diseases. Meat and milk are high sources of dietary phosphate. The approximate oral intake for a normal person is about 1000 mg out of which about 70% is absorbed. The kidneys excrete any excess phosphate and maintain the blood level. If excessive oral intake of phosphorus is combined with excessive vitamin D administration, severe hyperphosphatemia may occur. In patients with renal failure, phosphate cannot be excreted by the kidneys. Hyperphosphatemia associated with hypocalcemia is the characteristic blood abnormality in chronic renal failure.

Hypophosphatemia

It occurs when there is decreased phosphate absorption from the gut, increased renal excretion or when there is shift of phosphorus from ECF to the ICF. Decreased intake may occur in alcoholics or in those taking phosphate binder medicines (see the box).

Phosphate binders

The phosphate binders are tablets or powders which are **given with food** so that they bind with the phosphate in the diet and prevent the absorption by the intestine.

They help to prevent hyperphosphatemia in patients with renal failure.

Example: Aluminium hydroxide, calcium acetate/carbonate, sevelemer, and lanthanum carbonate.

In conditions like vitamin D deficiency, hyperparathyroidism, familial phosphate wasting or when using some drugs, the kidney fail to reabsorb phosphorus. Such patients may have neuromuscular symptoms, numbness, muscle weakness and anemia. Treatment is mainly by oral phosphate replacement. These patients may have hypokalemia and hypomagnesemia also and it should be corrected simultaneously.

DISORDERS OF MAGNESIUM METABOLISM

Magnesium is the fourth most abundant cation in the body. In the intracellular compartment, its concentration is higher. It has a very important role to play in intracellular enzyme systems and metabolism. Hypomagnesemia may predispose critically ill patients to a variety of life threatening complications. Body contains 21–28gm of Mg^{++}, nearly 70% is stored in the skeleton. The blood contains **1.6–2.0 mEq/L** (35% protein bound and 65% ionized) and the remaining is inside the cell. In times of stress, magnesium requirement of the body increases. Serum Mg level is maintained in a narrow range by the kidneys and GIT. Green vegetables, milk and meat are the important dietary sources of Mg^{++}.

Hypermagnesemia is when serum Mg level >3 mEq/L. The common causes are renal failure (due to defective excretion of Mg^{++}), severe pre-eclampsia, when IV magnesium sulfate is administered or following use of Mg^{++} or Mg^{++} containing drugs. During Mg^{++} infusion, serum level over 7 mEq/L may result in hypotension, drowsiness, coma, respiratory failure, cardiac arrhythmias, atrioventricular block and cardiac arrest. The ECG changes are almost similar to hyperkalemia.

For treatment, the primary disease/causative factor must be corrected. For severe hypermagnesmia, hemodialysis is done because, it will help to remove Mg^{++} from blood and reduce the symptoms.

Hypomagnesemia

Hypomagnesemia means low Mg level **(<1.2 mEq/L** in blood). It is a problem which may coexist with hypokalemia. If a patient suffering from hypokalemia and does not improve in spite of correction of potassium, associated Mg deficiency is suspected. Hypomagnesemia may occur in patients with diabetes mellitus due to loss from GIT and poor intake. The other causes are:

1. Loss from GIT (prolonged nasogastric aspiration/chronic diarrhea/pancreatitis)
2. Renal loss (diuretics/conditions of polyuria)
3. During correction of diabetic ketoacidosis
   Drugs (diuretics/anticancer drugs/immunosuppressive drugs/aminoglycosides)
4. Metastatic cancer

Magnesium supplements are to be given by mouth as magnesium salts (5 mg/kg/day) for mild to moderate magnesium deficiency. Renal failure is a contraindication for Mg^{++} administration. Magnesium infusions should be given in ICUs under close monitoring. Frequent monitoring of serum Mg^{++} level is necessary during IV Mg^{++} treatment. The knee jerk should be checked frequently. If the reflex becomes sluggish/absent or the respiratory rate decreases, it is a sign of toxic level and the infusion must be discontinued. Often hypomagnesmia co-exists with hypokalemia, hypocalcemia and metabolic acidosis.

31

Simplified Understanding of Acid–Base Balance

R Kasi Visweswaran

In this chapter, we will try to understand the primary acid–base disorder and the normal body compensations. The term **acidemia** means 'acid in blood' and **alkalemia** means 'alkali in blood'. The term acidosis and alkalosis are used for the disease conditions that produce acidemia and alkalemia.

Common investigation reports used in acid–base analysis are **pH, pCO$_2$ and HCO$_3$.**

The blood gas analyser or ABG machine is used for assessing the above. Most busy ICUs in major hospitals have the machine in the ICU itself. The machine measures the pH, pCO$_2$, electrolytes, oxygen saturation and calculates the HCO$_3$ and anion gap. It is also possible to estimate HCO$_3$ in a biochemistry laboratory.

a. The normal **pH of blood is 7.4** (range 7.35–7.45). The blood pH should be maintained in the narrow range. It is important that the body maintains proper (optimum) pH for maintenance of cellular functions. The blood pH is maintained with the help of 'Buffers'. Buffers are chemical systems which prevent immediate changes in the pH. The important buffers in the body are bicarbonate, phosphate, proteins, hemoglobin and bone (bicarbonate in bone). A **pH** of 7 is neutral. The lower the **pH,** the more acidic the **blood.** The diet, presence of vomiting (loss of acid), diarrhea (loss of alkali), abnormalities in lung function (by changing pCO$_2$), endocrine function, kidney function, and urinary tract infection can change the pH. We have studied about **pH** in school classes. pH is defined as the degree of acidity or basicity (alkalinity) of an aqueous solution and is expressed as a number. It is roughly the negative logarithm to base 10 of the concentration hydrogen ions or H$^+$ (as units/L).

1. $pH = \log_{10}$ of $\dfrac{\text{Base}}{\text{Acid}}$

For clinical purposes, we can consider that the pH is proportional to ($\propto$)

2. $pH \propto \dfrac{\text{Base}}{\text{Acid}}$

The base is HCO_3 and acid is carbonic acid H_2CO_3. Therefore,

3. $pH \propto \dfrac{HCO_3}{H_2CO_3}$

Since H_2CO_3 dissociates into CO_2 and H_2O, the formula can be rewritten as

4. $pH \propto \dfrac{HCO_3}{CO_2 + H_2O}$

CO_2 is measurable in blood as pCO_2. So, we take partial pressure of carbon dioxide in the blood (pCO_2) to represent the acid. Finally,

5. $pH \propto \dfrac{HCO_3}{pCO_2}$

We will use **this formula**—pH is proportional to HCO_3 divided by pCO_2 (for further discussion, see the box).

In any formula, if the numerator is increased or denominator is decreased, the value will go up. If the numerator is decreased or denominator increased, the value will go down.

Examples: Take the simple formula → $500/10 = 50$

If the numerator increases to 800   → $800/10 = 80$

If the denominator decreases to 5   → $500/5 = 100$

If the numerator decreases to 300   → $300/10 = 30$

If the denominator increases to 25   → $500/25 = 20$

The normal **pCO_2** is 40 mmHg. It may vary from 36 to 44 mmHg. When the breathing is inadequate, there is retention of CO_2 and the pCO_2 increases. If you apply increased pCO_2 in the formula, then

$$\downarrow pH \propto \dfrac{HCO_3}{\uparrow pCO_2}$$

the value of pH should come down—**low pH is acidosis**. Since the **primary change is in pCO_2, it is respiratory.** Therefore, a condition with primary increase in pCO_2 will result in **respiratory acidosis**.

When the person is overbreathing (hyperventilation), the CO_2 is removed from the body because of excessive respiration ('washed off') and the pCO_2 comes down. If you apply to pCO_2 in the equation, you will note that the value of pH will increase.

$$\uparrow pH \propto \frac{HCO_3}{\downarrow pCO_2}$$

High pH is alkalosis. Since the **primary change is in pCO_2, it is respiratory.** Therefore, a condition with primary decrease in pCO_2 will result in **respiratory alkalosis.**

The normal **HCO_3 is 24 mmol/L or mEq/L.** It may vary from 22 to 26 mmol/L. When body produces more acid or when kidneys are not excreting the acid, the bicarbonate will act as a buffer to neutralize the acid. So, the level of bicarbonate will come down (see the box).

- Body produces about 1 mmol/kg body weight of H^+ ions a day from metabolism of food.
- The kidney excretes approximately 1 mmol/kg/day of H^+ ions
- For every H^+ ion excreted, the body gains one bicarbonate.
- Every 1 mEq bicarbonate administered neutralises one H^+ ion.

Any primary change in HCO_3 is metabolic: If more acid is produced or if acid is not excreted, the HCO_3 comes down. When HCO_3 comes down, the pH also comes down. So, pH is **metabolic acidosis.**

$$\downarrow pH \propto \frac{\downarrow HCO_3}{pCO_2}$$

In metabolic alkalosis, there is primary increase in HCO_3. Therefore, the pH also increases. Since the primary change is in HCO_3, it is metabolic and since the pH is high, it is alkalosis. Therefore, conditions with primary increase in HCO_3 cause **metabolic alkalosis.**

Thus, there are 4 primary acid–base disorders.

If the primary change is in bicarbonate, the disorder is metabolic.
If the primary change is in pCO_2, the disorder is respiratory.

Primary **fall in bicarbonate:** **Metabolic acidosis**
Primary **rise in bicarbonate:** **Metabolic alkalosis**
Primary **fall in pCO₂:**   **Respiratory alkalosis**
Primary **rise in pCO₂:**   **Respiratory acidosis**

In the clinical pH equation, watch the direction of the arrows in the four primary acid–base disorders.

$\downarrow pH \propto \dfrac{\downarrow HCO_3}{pCO_2}$ Metabolic acidosis. Primay disturbance is fall in HCO_3	$\uparrow pH \propto \dfrac{\uparrow HCO_3}{pCO_2}$ Metabolic alkalosis. Primay disturbance is rise in HCO_3
$\downarrow pH \propto \dfrac{HCO_3}{\uparrow pCO_2}$ Respiratory acidosis. Primay disturbance is rise in pCO_2 ($PaCO_2$)	$\uparrow pH \propto \dfrac{HCO_3}{\downarrow pCO_2}$ Respiratory alkalosis. Primay disturbance is fall in pCO_2 ($PaCO_2$)

COMMON ACID–BASE DISORDERS

We have seen that acidosis can occur when

1. Acids are added to the body from outside (exogenous)
2. Acids are added to the body from inside (endogenous)
3. Alkali is lost from the body (loss of bicarbonate containing fluid)
4. Failure to produce enough bicarbonate in the body.
5. Excessive carbon dioxide accumulates in the blood.

Similarly, alkalosis can occur when

1. Alkalis are added to the body from outside (exogenous), e.g. sodium bicarbonate
2. Alkalis are added to the body from inside (endogenous)
3. Acid is lost from the body (loss of gastric acid due to vomiting)
4. Excessive carbon dioxide is removed from blood

Anion Gap

Anion gap (AG) is used to analyse metabolic acidosis. In blood, for every anion, there is a cation and there is no actual gap. For calculating the AG, only Na^+ is considered in the cationic side and $Cl^- + HCO_3$ in the anionic side. Other measured and unmeasured anions and cations are excluded from the equation. AG is calculated from serum sodium, chloride and bicarbonate as follows.

$$AG = Na^+ - (Cl^- + HCO_3)$$

Normally the difference between them is about 12 ± 4.

Example: If $Na^+ = 140$ mEq/L
$Cl^- = 106$ mEq/L and
$HCO_3^- = 24$ mEq/L

Anion gap is calculated as

$$AG = 140 - (106 + 24) = 140 - 130 = 10 \text{ (normal range)}$$

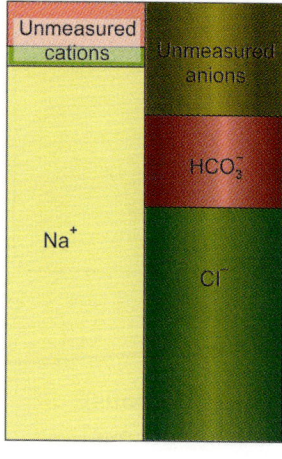
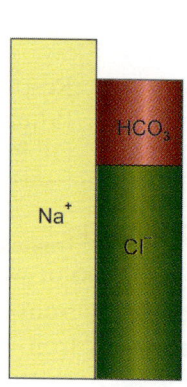

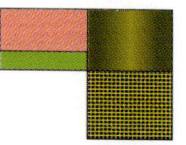
The shaded area represents anion gap

METABOLIC ACIDOSIS

Metabolic acidosis is classified mainly as high anion gap and normal anion gap.

High anion gap metabolic acidosis occurs due to:

1. *Due to addition of endogenous acids:* Ketoacidosis in uncontrolled diabetes/starvation and alcoholism and uremia (accumulation of waste products in renal failure).
2. *Due to accumulation of lactic acid:* Shock, drugs, liver disease, uremia.
3. *Due to addition of exogenous acids:* Methanol, ethylene, glycol, formic acid, salicylate poisoning.

Normal anion gap metabolic acidosis occurs in:

4. Bicarbonate loss due to diarrhea, enterocutaneous fistula and ureterosigmoidostomy.
5. Loss of bicarbonate through kidney—proximal/distal renal tubular acidosis (defective H^+ ion secretion in kidney)
6. Ammonium chloride (acid) ingestion.

METABOLIC ALKALOSIS

Metabolic alkalosis occurs commonly in the wards with very sick patients and in ICUs. It can occur as a result of loss of gastric hydrochloric acid due to vomiting or continuous nasogastric suction. It may also result due to loss of chloride through the kidneys following diuretic use. Measurement of urine chloride excretion helps to classify the causes as "chloride responsive" and "chloride resistant" metabolic alkalosis. Conditions associated with dehydration are chloride responsive and respond well to treatment with normal saline infusions. (Normal saline is sodium chloride 0.9 gm % concentration.) Chloride resistant metabolic alkalosis occurs in some inherited kidney diseases, hypokalemia or when there is excessive mineralocorticoid hormone.

RESPIRATORY ACIDOSIS

Respiratory acidosis is primary elevation in $PaCO_2$ (hypercapnia). There is reduction in pH. CO_2 accumulates when CO_2 production is more than CO_2 excretion by the lung. These are:

1. Depression of respiratory center (sedation, hypnotics, anesthetic agents, cerebrovascular accidents, central nervous system infection)
2. Weakness of respiratory muscles (myopathy, myasthenia gravis, Guillain-Barré syndrome, hypokalemia)
3. Airway obstructions (mechanical, asthma)
4. Alveolar diseases (bronchopneumonia, ARDS, pulmonary edema or COPD, obesity and hypoventilation), or
5. Diminished ventilation due to rib fracture, pneumothorax or lung collapse or aspiration.

The major treatment is to clear the airway, provide oxygen and mechanical support, if necessary. Oxygen should be administered carefully because, in chronic hypercapnia, oxygen administration may further depress the respiratory center and worsen hypercapnia. If chronic hypercapnia is corrected suddenly with mechanical ventilation, the patient may develop a more serious condition called posthypercapnic alkalosis.

RESPIRATORY ALKALOSIS

In respiratory alkalosis there is low pCO_2 (hypocapnia). When the patient is hyperventilating (overbreathing), thereby washing out the CO_2 from blood. It can occur in people with extreme anxiety, hysteria, pain or during normal pregnancy. It occurs in those with sepsis, hepatic failure, brain tumor, pulmonary embolism, salicylate intoxication and following rapid correction of metabolic acidosis.

In addition to identifying the underlying cause, O_2 administration helps to improve hyperventilation. If there is no oxygen deficiency (sPO_2 is normal), the patient is reassured and asked to re-breath into a paper bag to correct this acid–base abnormality.

Collecting Blood Sample for ABG

Collection of blood sample for arterial blood gas (ABG) analysis is by puncturing the artery and great care should be exercised.

   a. If radial artery is punctured, Allen's test must be performed to confirm the integrity of the ulnar artery and palmar arch.
   b. Femoral or brachial artery may also be used.
   c. Meticulous sterile precautions must be followed.
   d. Blood from the artery should not be aspirated but must flow directly into the heparinised syringe.
   e. The syringe should have low friction and a smoothly moving piston.
   f. Contact of the blood sample with air should be avoided since it may give wrong results.
   g. The sample is labeled and sent for analysis immediately.
   h. ABG should be done in emergency or critical condition in an unstable patient or those on ventilator.
   i. It should not be used as a 'routine' investigation.

Main data obtained from ABG are **pH, pCO_2 and HCO_3**. These are used mainly in the interpretation of acid–base status.

Normal pH	– 7.4	(range 7.35–7.45)
Normal HCO_3	– 24 mmol/L	(range 22–26 mmol/L)
Normal pCO_2	– 40 mmHg	(range 35–45 mmHg)

Steps in Interpretation

Step 1: Check if pH, pCO_2 and HCO_3 are in normal range. If they are normal, there may be no acid–base disorder. But in a critically ill patient, with multiple problems, it may suggest that the person may have a complicated double or triple acid–base disorder.

Step 2: If pH <7.35, patient has acidemia. It may be due to either metabolic acidosis (when the bicarbonate is lower) or respiratory acidosis (in which case, the $PaCO_2$ will be high).

If pH >7.45, patient has alkalemia. It may be due to either metabolic alkalosis (when the bicarbonate is higher) or respiratory alkalosis (in which case, the $PaCO_2$ will be low).

Example 1: pH = 7.30, HCO_3 = 18 mmol/L, pCO_2 = 38 mmHg

pH	= 7.30	→ acidemia	
HCO_3	= 18	→ (low) metabolic	
pCO_2	= 38	→ normal range	∴ **Metabolic acidosis**

Example 2: pH = 7.30, HCO_3 = 24 mmol/L, pCO_2 = 66 mmHg

pH	= 7.30	→ acidemia	
HCO_3	= 24	→ normal range	
pCO_2	= 66	→ (high) respiratory	∴ **Respiratory acidosis**

Example 3: pH = 7.51, HCO_3 = 31 mmol/L, pCO_2 = 42 mmHg

pH	= 7.51	→ alkalemia	
HCO_3	= 31	→ (high) metabolic	
pCO_2	= 42	→ normal range	∴ **Metabolic alkalosis**

Example 4: pH = 7.48, HCO_3 = 25 mmol/L, pCO_2 = 28 mmHg

pH	= 7.48	→ alkalemia	
HCO_3	= 26	→ normal range	
pCO_2	= 28	→ (low) respiratory	∴ **Respiratory alkalosis**

The body tries to compensate for the primary acid–base disorder with a view to normalize the pH. If the numerator and denominator move in the same direction, the value of the formula does not change (see the box).

In any formula, if both the numerator and the denominator are decreased or both are increased, the value does not change significantly.

Example: Take the simple formula   → 500/10 = 50
If the numerator and denominator **increase** to 800 and 16   → 800/16 = 50 or
If the numerator and denominator **decrease** to 250 and 5   → 250/5 = 50

The compensatory mechanisms in the body are designed to increase or decrease the numerator or denominator depending on the direction of the other. This is called the 'same direction rule'.

$$pH \propto \frac{HCO_3}{pCO_2}$$

In the above equation, according to the 'same direction rule' of compensation, if there is lowering or ($\downarrow$) HCO_3 (metabolic acidosis), the normal compensation should be ($\downarrow$) pCO_2 (respiratory alkalosis).

The compensation for the four primary acid–base disorders is shown as follows:

Primary disorders	Compensation
a. Metabolic acidosis ($\downarrow HCO_3$)	Respiratory alkalosis ($\downarrow pCO_2$)
b. Metabolic alkalosis ($\uparrow HCO_3$)	Respiratory acidosis ($\uparrow pCO_2$)
c. Respiratory acidosis ($\uparrow pCO_2$)	Metabolic alkalosis ($\uparrow HCO_3$)
d. Respiratory alkalosis ($\downarrow pCO_2$)	Metabolic acidosis ($\downarrow HCO_3$)

Obeying and disobeying the 'same direction rule'

In a primary acid–base disorder, the compensatory shift of the numerator and denominator will be in the same direction.

So, if the numerator and denominator in the fraction move in the same direction, the compensation is normal.

If the numerator and denominator in the equation move in the opposite directions, it is not the normal body compensation. It may mean two or more disorders.

Example 5: pH = 7.55, HCO_3 = 40 mmol/L, pCO_2 = 22 mmHg

(Direction of changes shown below. The arrow is upwards in the numerator and downward in the denominator.)

pH   = 7.55   →   Alkalemia
HCO_3 = 40   →   (High) metabolic
pCO_2 = 22   →   (Unexpectedly low) respiratory

See the direction of changes.

$$pH \propto \frac{HCO_3}{pCO_2} = \frac{\uparrow 40}{\downarrow 22} \quad \therefore \uparrow pH$$

Please note that the same direction rule is not followed in the example above. Therefore, it is not a simple acid–base disorder. According to the same direction rule, pCO_2 should have been high.

∴ **Metabolic alkalosis and respiratory alkalosis.**

There is also a limit up to which the compensation mechanisms work. If the compensation is too little or too much, it is often due to an associated disorder. The same direction rule also helps to identify such situations.

Two or three acid–base disorders in the same patient at the same time. A few examples of double acid–base commonly encountered in the wards are given below:

1. **Hyperemesis gravidarum: Metabolic alkalosis** due to vomiting and loss of acid + **respiratory alkalosis** due to hyperventilation in pregnancy.
2. **Severe vomiting with high fever: Metabolic alkalosis** due to vomiting, **respiratory alkalosis** due to fever, endotoxemia and hyperventilation.
3. **Salicylate overdose: Metabolic acidosis** due to acid (salicylate) load and **respiratory alkalosis** due to stimulation of respiratory center and hyperventilation.
4. **Chronic obstructive pulmonary disease (COPD) + vomiting: Respiratory acidosis** due to COPD, **metabolic alkalosis** due to vomiting.
5. **COPD + Diuretic use: Respiratory acidosis** due to COPD, **metabolic alkalosis** due to diuretic.
6. **Uremia with vomiting: Metabolic acidosis** due to uremia, **metabolic alkalosis** due to vomiting.
7. **Diabetics ketosis with vomiting: Metabolic acidosis** due to ketoacidosis, **metabolic alkalosis** due to vomiting.

By systematically analyzing the ABG report, it will be possible to understand the primary acid–base disorder, find out if the compensation of the body is adequate and suspect if more than one disorders are present in the same patient.

Index

H

Hairloss 99
half and half nails 83
Half normal saline with 5%
    dextrose (1/2 NS-D5) 215
Hansen's disease 91
Hay's test 50
HELLP syndrome 103
Hematuria 29
Hemodialysis 168
Hemofilter 172
Hemofiltration 177
Hemoglobin 55
Hemolytic uremic syndrome
    41, 103
Hemorrhagic cystitis 99
Henoch-Schönlein purpura
    (HSP) 86
Hepatitis B surface antigen
    (HbsAg) 59
Hepatorenal syndrome 102
Hesitancy 82
High anion gap metabolic
    acidosis 240
Hilum 5
HIV 91
    screening test 59
Homogentisic acid 49
Horseshoe kidneys 25
Human
    albumin 218
    eucocyte antigen (HLA) typing 60
    Organ Transplantation Act in
        1994 178
Hyaline casts 54
Hydroxyethyl starch 219
Hyperacute rejection 184
Hypercalcemia 232
Hypercalciuria 117
Hypercholesterolemia 30, 59
Hyperemesis gravidarum 245
Hyperkalemia 21
Hyperlipidemia 59
Hypermagnesemia 235
Hypernatremia 222, 227
Hyperoxaluria 117

Hyperparathyroidism 83, 117
Hyperphosphatemia 234
Hypertension 30, 38, 84
Hypertensive
    emergencies 140
    encephalopathy 33, 85
Hypertonic sodium chloride
    (3% NaCl) 217
Hypertriglyceridemia 59
Hyperuricosuria 117
Hypervolemia 221
Hypervolemic
    hypernatremia 226
    hyponatremia 224
Hypoalbuminemia 30
Hypocalcemia 232
Hypokalemia 21
Hypomagnesemia 235
Hyponatremia 21, 221
Hypophosphatasia 58
Hypophosphatemia 58, 234
Hypophosphatemic rickets 37
Hypoplasia/dysplasia 40
Hypotension 98
Hypovolemia 221
Hypovolemic
    hypernatremia 226
    hyponatremia 224

I

IgA 58
IgD 58
IgE 58
IgG 58
IgM 58
Immune-electrophoresis 58
Immunoglobulins (Igs) 58
Immunosuppression 31
Incontinence 82
Indeterminate metabolic
    'activity' 120
Inferior 5
Infertility 83, 99
Infrequently relapsing NS 32
Interleukin-2 receptor
    antagonists 184